DISABILITY AND THE

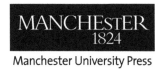

Manchester University Press

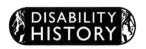

Series editors

Dr Julie Anderson, Professor Walton O. Schalick, III

This series published by Manchester University Press responds to the growing interest in disability as a discipline worthy of historical research. The series has a broad international historical remit, encompassing issues that include class, race, gender, age, war, medical treatment, professionalisation, environments, work, institutions and cultural and social aspects of disablement including representations of disabled people in literature, film, art and the media.

Already published
Deafness, community and culture in Britain: leisure and cohesion, 1945-1995
Martin Atherton
Rethinking modern prostheses in Anglo-American commodity cultures, 1820–1939
Claire L. Jones (ed.)
Destigmatising mental illness? Professional politics and public education in Britain, 1870–1970
Vicky Long
Intellectual disability: a conceptual history, 1200–1900
Patrick McDonagh, C. F. Goodey and Tim Stainton (eds)
Fools and idiots? Intellectual disability in the Middle Ages
Irina Metzler
Framing the moron: the social construction of feeble-mindedness in the American eugenics era
Gerald V. O'Brien
Recycling the disabled: army, medicine, and modernity in WWI Germany
Heather R. Perry
Disability in the Industrial Revolution: physical impairment in British coalmining, 1780–1880
David M. Turner and Daniel Blackie
Worth saving: disabled children during the Second World War
Sue Wheatcroft

DISABILITY AND THE VICTORIANS

ATTITUDES, INTERVENTIONS, LEGACIES

Edited by Iain Hutchison, Martin Atherton and
Jaipreet Virdi

Manchester University Press

Published by Manchester University Press
Oxford Road, Manchester M13 9PL

www.manchesteruniversitypress.co.uk

British Library Cataloguing-in-Publication Data
A catalogue record for this book is available from the British Library

ISBN   978 1 5261 4571 0   hardback
ISBN   978 1 5261 6392 9   paperback

First published 2020
Paperback published 2022

The publisher has no responsibility for the persistence or accuracy of URLs for any external or third-party internet websites referred to in this book, and does not guarantee that any content on such websites is, or will remain, accurate or appropriate.

Typeset
by Toppan Best-set Premedia Limited

In memory of Mike Oliver and Anne Borsay

Contents

List of illustrations   *page* viii

List of contributors   ix

Series editors' foreword   xi

Foreword – *Karen A. Sayer*   xii

Introduction – *Iain Hutchison, Martin Atherton and Jaipreet Virdi*   1

Part I: Attitudes

1   Restoration to usefulness: Victorian middle-class attitudes towards
    the healthcare of the working poor – *Amy W. Farnbach Pearson*   21

2   Imperial lives: confronting the legacies of empire, disability
    and the Victorians – *Esme Cleall*   38

3   Disabling the author in mid-Victorian realist fiction: case
    studies of George Eliot and Harriet Martineau – *Deborah M. Fratz*   55

Part II: Interventions

4   Medicalising deafness in Victorian London: the Royal Ear
    Hospital, 1816–1900 – *Jaipreet Virdi*   73

5   Drunkenness, degeneration and disability in England
    – *Joanne Woiak*   92

6   Victorian medical awareness of childhood language disabilities
    – *Paula Hellal and Marjorie Lorch*   110

7   'Happiness and usefulness increased': consuming ability in the
    antebellum artificial limb market – *Caroline Lieffers*   126

Part III: Legacies

8   The disabled child in an industrial metropolis: Glasgow's
    children's hospital, Scottish convalescent homes 'in the country'
    and East Park Home for Infirm Children – *Iain Hutchison*   145

9   *The Panopticon*: towards an intimate history of special schools
    for the blind – *Fred Reid*   164

10 Allowed to be idle: perpetuating Victorian attitudes to
    deafness and employability in United Kingdom social policy
    – *Martin Atherton*   177

Index   195

Illustrations

4.1   Selina Hewitt, Mary Ann Hauge and Mary Haines, allegedly
      'successfully cured' at the Royal Dispensary for Diseases of
      the Ear. From: John Harrison Curtis, *An Essay on the
      Deaf and Dumb*, 2nd edn (London: Longman, 1834).
      Reproduced by permission of Yale University, Harvey
      Cushing/John Hay Whitney Medical Library.   *page* 80
7.1   Illustration for Palmer's patent legs. From: *The Bane and
      Antidote: A Surgical Adjuvant and Reporter of Artificial
      Limbs*, ed. Frank Palmer, No. 8 (January 1859), p. 35.
      Reproduced by permission of the National Library of
      Medicine, US Department of Health and Human Services.   133
8.1   Children at the RHSC Country Branch. From the private
      collection of Elizabeth Anderson.   150
8.2   East Park Home boys, late 1880s. From the private collection
      of Iain Hutchison.   155

Contributors

Martin Atherton (co-editor) is a social historian of deafness and deaf people. His research covers a range of topics, including lived experiences and narratives, leisure and sport, education, family relationships and social policy. Martin retired from his position in the School of Humanities and Social Sciences at the University of Central Lancashire in summer 2018.

Esme Cleall is a lecturer in the Department of History, University of Sheffield and is a social and cultural historian of the British Empire. Her work explores the relationship between ethnicity, religion, gender and disability across different sites of the nineteenth- and twentieth-century British Empire, including India, southern Africa and imperial Britain. Her first book, *Missionary Discourses of Difference*, was published with Palgrave in 2012 and she has since produced several articles on disability and deafness.

Deborah M. Fratz is Associate Professor of English, Languages and Literatures at the University of Wisconsin-Whitewater. She teaches nineteenth-century British literature and critical writing and has a particular interest in the representation of disability in Romanticism literature.

Paula Hellal is Honorary Research Fellow in the Department of Applied Linguistics and Communication, Birkbeck College, University of London. She has published extensively on childhood language development and disabilities, and has a particular interest in nineteenth-century responses and attitudes.

Iain Hutchison (co-editor) is a Research Associate at the Centre for the History of Medicine at the University of Glasgow and a board member of the Disability History Association. His main research interests concern the experience of mental, physical and sensory disability in Scotland across the long nineteenth century.

Caroline Lieffers is an Assistant Professor of History at The King's University, Edmonton, Canada. She specialises in disability, health technologies and transnational exchange in the nineteenth and early twentieth centuries.

Marjorie Lorch is Professor of Neurolinguistics in the Department of Applied Linguistics and Communication, Birkbeck College, University of London. She researches how language is organised in the brain through the investigation of neurogenic language and communication disorders. One strand of her research focuses on the nineteenth-century history of ideas about language and communication and its relation to thought.

Amy W. Farnbach Pearson is a historical anthropologist at the Health Sciences Center, University of New Mexico and a Research Affiliate at the Center for Bioarchaeological Research, Arizona State University. She investigates Western medical concepts of health and disease and doctor–patient relationships.

Fred Reid is Honorary Professor in History at the University of Warwick. His research interests are various, including British labour history, history and literature, and all aspects of blindness. He himself became blind at the age of fourteen. As well as his academic work, he has served as President of the National Federation of the Blind, as a trustee of the Royal National Institute of Blind People and on the executive boards of the Disability Income Group and the Disability Alliance.

Jaipreet Virdi (co-editor) is Assistant Professor in the Department of History, University of Delaware. Her work intersects the history of medicine and disability history. Her first book is *Hearing Happiness: Fakes, Frauds, and Fads in Deafness Cures* (University of Chicago Press).

Joanne Woiak is a lecturer in the Department of Disability Studies, University of Washington. Her research interests encompass the social justice implications of knowledge about genetics, reproduction and health in the modern era. She focuses on disability in American and British history and culture, including the history of eugenics and sterilisation, discourses about alcoholism, science fiction and disability pedagogy.

Series editors' foreword

You know a subject has achieved maturity when a book series is dedicated to it. In the case of disability, while it has co-existed with human beings for centuries the study of disability's history is still quite young.

In setting up this series, we chose to encourage multi-methodologic history rather than a purely traditional historical approach, as researchers in disability history come from a wide variety of disciplinary backgrounds. Equally, 'disability' history is a diverse topic which benefits from a variety of approaches in order to appreciate its multi-dimensional characteristics.

A test for the team of authors and editors who bring you this series is typical of most series, but disability also brings other consequential challenges. At this time disability is highly contested as a social category in both developing and developed contexts. Inclusion, philosophy, money, education, visibility, sexuality, identity and exclusion are but a handful of the social categories in play. With this degree of politicisation, language is necessarily a cardinal focus.

In an effort to support the plurality of historical voices, the editors have elected to give fair rein to language. Language is historically contingent, and can appear offensive to our contemporary sensitivities. The authors and editors believe that the use of terminology that accurately reflects the historical period of any book in the series will assist readers in their understanding of the history of disability in time and place.

Finally, disability offers the cultural, social and intellectual historian a new 'take' on the world we know. We see disability history as one of a few nascent fields with the potential to reposition our understanding of the flow of cultures, society, institutions, ideas and lived experience. Conceptualisations of 'society' since the early modern period have heavily stressed principles of autonomy, rationality and the subjectivity of the individual agent. Consequently we are frequently oblivious to the historical contingency of the present with respect to those elements. Disability disturbs those foundational features of 'the modern.' Studying disability history helps us resituate our policies, our beliefs and our experiences.

Julie Anderson
Walton O. Schalick, III

Foreword

The conference 'Disability and the Victorians – Confronting Legacies', from which this book took root, was held in 2012 under the auspices of the Leeds Centre for Victorian Studies (LCVS). It was the first international conference to bring Victorian Studies and disability history together. Founded in 1994, the now nationally and internationally recognised LCVS was established at Leeds Trinity University (known as Leeds Trinity and All Saints College at the point of the Centre's foundation). It was set up by academics working in history, English, philosophy, theology and religious studies who were determined to work across, between and around disciplines in order to think, not just about the Victorians in the confines of the nineteenth century, but also about what the 'Victorians' have come to mean in the longer term: their cultural, social and political impact, nationally and internationally, in the time since Queen Victoria's death in 1901.

A conference that set out to address the legacies emerging from the Victorian period when it came to the experience and the cultural conceptualisation of disability was therefore always going to be important for the LCVS. The aim was to mesh Victorian Studies and Disability Studies: two truly interdisciplinary fields of enquiry. However, when LCVS initially imagined the event, those of us who led it and had the passion to see it through to its conclusion knew that Victorian Studies as a field had to actively 'confront' the legacies of that period. The conference had to speak back to the attitudes, interventions, taxonomies, institutions and other traces of the Victorian past that have so often shaped 'disability' since that period, but which have also shaped disciplinary boundaries. In order to do this, the conference could not be planned, organised or run without the experience and expertise of disabled stakeholders.

At the most fundamental planning level, and at the conceptual level of 'being' a scholar/in the academy, it was very clear that a long lead-in time was going to be needed to 'hack' the campus. We therefore formed a conference-organising committee in 2010 that included myself as conference lead and two other colleagues linked to LCVS – its current Director, Dr Nathan Uglow, and Dr Susan Anderson, who also researches in earlier periods and performance – administrators Joy Hamblin and Julie Wadsworth, and the University's Dyslexia and Disability Co-ordinator, Deborah Altman, who worked in Student Services.

Deborah was a vital addition: she not only knew the buildings and facilities that we already had, because she had had to write them up for students at all levels and run the Disabled Students network, but she also knew what we were missing. She suspected, rightly, that there would be additional considerations; and she knew that she 'didn't know what she didn't know'. Through her we reached out to local stakeholders via DIAL LEEDS Ltd, a disabled people's user-led organisation founded in 1979. And, through our pooled networks, also brought in CoHearentVision – at that point the working title of the Leeds Society for Deaf and Blind People, established in 1876 – and Jill Jones from DEX (Deaf Ex-Mainstreamers, based in Leeds). That stakeholder group, paid for by the University, was crucial in making the conference work across the buildings and across the scheduling, and bringing the whole thing alive. We academics held the line in rejecting or seeking revisions to proposals for papers that treated 'disability' as a metaphor, as anything less than a historically lived experience, but it was the stakeholder group that made this a landmark event.

Delegates of all career stages came from Nigeria, Canada, the United States, Australia, the continent of Europe and the UK, and included leading authors such as Martha Stoddard Holmes, author of *Fictions of Affliction: Physical Disability in Victorian Culture* (2009), in the then emerging sub-discipline of cultural Disability Studies. But, because of the stakeholder group, the conference was also busy with stands, videos and 'pop-up' posters being presented by activists, local groups, heritage providers, British Sign Language interpreters and second-hand bookstalls. There were community projects, such as the Heritage Lottery-funded Deaf History Project (since concluded) based at Bradford Talking Media, as well as presentations by leading campaigners, including John Hay MBE, Chair of the British Deaf History Society.[1] We had a 'field visit' to the Thackray Medical Museum, where delegates were given guided tours, were able to handle objects in the collection and saw the newly accessioned 100-year-old testimony in hand-sewn textile of Lorina Butler.[2]

The success of this field visit was due, in no small part, to the stakeholder group, which had pre-paid 'big enough' taxis, rather than just a bus, funded by the British Association of Victorian Studies. Thanks to the group, we had a quiet space for rest and relaxation away from the wider conference bustle; a set of instructions about how to navigate a campus that included an appreciation of the 'uphill' walk from the local railway station; booked campus residence rooms that had good accessibility (turning circles, hoists available if needed, etc.); a high-contrast map of the campus and its accessible routes; lighting that did not flicker and that the hearing loop worked, with technical support on standby; lapel and lectern microphones for speakers and hand-held microphones for the question and answer sessions; a designated place for assistance dogs to 'go' during their scheduled breaks; detailed instructions for the chairs of panels (e.g. about repeating questions and running to time); lots of absolutely vital, paid student 'runners'; specialist cutlery and straws available in the dining room;

and a schedule that had 'proper' breaks between sessions to move easefully from room to room and have time to eat, drink and talk. The value of the long breaks for networking, rest, collaboration and fuelling up on ideas and food became a lasting legacy in their own right and something that many academic presenters took away with them.

Some of the things we did, we chose to do, almost spontaneously, as acts of hospitality and welcome. A couple of delegates could come only if they brought their children, so the children got their own delegate packs with badges, notepads, colouring pens and stickers: they were utterly delighted! The receptionists had boxes of basic supplies on standby – the sorts of things that people forget to pack, such as toiletries – to save those who needed them the hassle of getting to the shops. Because the campus is out of town, we also decided to have evening entertainment. Our cabaret included deaf comedian John Smith of *Beautiful BSL*, and comedian Lee Ridley, aka Lost Voice Guy, a man who has since won *Britain's Got Talent*!

In the years since the conference, the field has grown. Other meetings, and those working in other periods, have taken up the theme and run with it, adding, as Susan Anderson has observed, more nuance to our understanding of the ways in which disability has been thought of historically, and how we come/ are able to see it from our own standpoint in time.[3] But, for me, the conference out of which this book emerged has remained a turning point during which I learned not only about the Victorians, but – much more importantly – how to 'hack' a campus. I am sure that there are better approaches than those we adopted (but thank you to those who asked that I share what we did), and I am sure that it is necessary to hard-wire it in, legally and in policy-making, given that in 2016 the United Nations criticised the UK for disability rights violations, in part for stereotyping. But I also remember the new ways that people talked, created and worked *together* in the space of the event. That seems as important as ever. This collection carries forward those voices.

This post-event collection brings the fields of Victorian Studies and Disability Studies together, and it gives new momentum to the power generated by the conference. Since the LCVS was founded in 1994, Victorian Studies has changed from a field of enquiry that prioritised the exploration of interdisciplinarity, to acting as an interdisciplinary field that enquires about time. Within debates about periodisation – 'the long nineteenth century' versus the 'monarchical' 1837–1901 – questions about the temporal longevity of 'the Victorian' and the geographical locatedness of the Victorians have been constantly to the fore, even when the critique has been more cultural than historical. Today, the aesthetics of the Victorians shape the lives of the neo-Victorians who choose to make and remake the past in the present, and have been brought into the frame for academic analysis to disrupt, reconsider and sometimes reimagine the nineteenth century's 'dreaming into the future'. Yet, the field demonstrates that the work of thinking about the Victorians has always been more about those who are writing (the present) than about the Victorians (the past).[4]

What Disability Studies does, by remaining centred politically on the present, is sharpen and focus these habits of thought. Of course, Disability Studies has itself changed since its foundation within mid- to late twentieth-century disability activism. Much of this addresses the definition and reach of 'disability'. Here we have the ongoing discussion of the medical and social models, and then there are the debates about categories and hierarchies, belonging and refusal to belong (for example, the rejection of 'disabled' by the culturally rich deaf community, despite the legal categories), and on the impacts of changing metaphors and images of 'disability', etc.[5] Yet, what Disability Studies still does, and does to the benefit of Victorian Studies, is to generate an incisive, biting reminder that when we talk of the legacies of the Victorians after 1901, those legacies have had and still have a bearing on life as it is lived. Both fields now talk to each other much more than in 2010–12, and scholars publish across the journals of research in both fields.

By bringing the two fields together, what *Disability and the Victorians* does is demonstrate that it is essential to remain aware both of periodisation and time (i.e. that 'disability' is historically situated) and of the reality that, over a century later, this period can still appear in the contours of people's lives (across a geographic range that is itself a legacy of the Victorian). It shows us that we must engage in nuanced readings of the sources – archival records, artefacts, images, buildings – that we inherit from the nineteenth century, informed by knowledge of the past, framed by historically situated debates about, and understandings of, themes such as class, sex, 'race' and theology; elastic themes that changed over the period. But also, that those same sources can be traced to the present. They remain influential: unknowingly, in acceptance or in resistance, the Victorians have been implicated continuously in the framing and reframing of the social, economic, political, medical and experiential spaces of present 'disability'.

The Victorians have shaped, and continue to shape, the actual through their attitudes, interventions and legacies. The logical conclusion is that, by sculpting our lives, as this book shows, the Victorians also shape what we bring to bear as we seek them out to reimagine and reconstruct their past and the pasts of the lives that went, at the time, unnoticed, unconsidered and unaccounted.

Karen A. Sayer
Professor of Social and Cultural History
Leeds Trinity University

Notes

1 All materials from the project have since been deposited with the Yorkshire Film Archive, access via Deaf History Project, https://www.btm.org.uk/our-teams/deaf-history-project/, accessed 15 March 2019).

2 Another scroll stitched by Lorina Butler is in Norwich Castle Museum, http://norfolkmuseumscollections.org/#!/collections/search?q=lorina%2Bbulwer.

3 S. Anderson, *Historical Periodisation and Disability Studies*, blog written for Leeds Centre for Victoria Studies, 2015, www.leedstrinity.ac.uk/blogs/leeds-centre-for-victorian-studies/historical-periodisation-and-disability-studies.

4 Thanks to Professor Miles Taylor for his discussion of the meanings of 'Victorian' in 'Victorian Studies' at his Public Lecture and Workshop as Honorary Visiting Professor to the LCVS, Leeds Trinity University, 20 March 2019. Also, see Neo-Victorian Studies, http://neovictorianstudies.com/, accessed 22 March 2019.

5 *Disability Studies Quarterly*, http://dsq-sds.org/index, accessed 22 March 2019; *Journal of Literary and Cultural Disability Studies*, https://online.liverpooluniversitypress.co.uk/loi/jlcds.

INTRODUCTION

Iain Hutchison, Martin Atherton and Jaipreet Virdi

Disability and the Victorians: Attitudes, interventions, legacies brings together the work of eleven scholars. The collection focuses on the history of disability and, while showcasing the work of a diverse gathering of historians, it also gives a flavour of how disability history engages the work of scholars from other disciplines and how they, in turn, enhance historical thought and understanding. Equally, while the focus is on the Victorian era, a time during which society changed significantly, both at the bottom and from the top, it was also a time in which patterns developed that were to have an enduring influence. Therefore a taste of that enduring influence is presented in chapters that suggest the resilience of Victorian thought and practices in the modern era. Consequently, an underlying aim is to encourage readers to take a broad view, both of 'disability' and of Victorian influences and values.

'Disability' is a wide and multifaceted concept. Indeed, the thinking and actions of Victorian elites drew heavily on a whole range of ways of classifying, not only sections within society, but also behaviours that they considered to be socially and morally deviant. Yet the collective and all-embracing term 'disability' is a modern construct that only rarely appeared in their rhetoric. Notably, through the application of Poor Laws in England and Wales, Scotland, Ireland and beyond, what Victorians were guided by were their perceptions of able-bodiedness and ability to perform productive and self-supporting work, on the one hand, and, on the other, their judgement, in sometimes considerably divergent and subjective ways, of people who were disabled from working through a range of physical, sensory and mental impediments.[1] After all, the comfortable classes, charged with funding Poor Law provision, had a vested interest in reducing the numbers claiming poor relief.[2] As a consequence, they increasingly tried to differentiate between people whom they considered to be worthy of aid – people genuinely disabled from working, due to an impairment – and people whom they deemed to be unworthy of assistance and support, whom they considered to be able-bodied and capable of working, but who were unable or unwilling to find employment.[3]

The Victorian era, encompassing the latter six decades of the nineteenth century, was a period by which significant areas of the British Isles had become industrialised and urbanised. Both processes exacerbated the extent of impairing conditions, these ranging from industrial injury resulting from employment in mills, factories, quarries and collieries and on the burgeoning railways, through to the prevalence of debilitating physiological illnesses. These included diseases, such as tuberculosis and rickets, that were aggravated by squalid, overcrowded housing conditions, poor sanitation and uncontrolled industrial pollution. Maria Frawley points out that the Victorians were not only dealing with the consequences of rapid industrialisation, but simultaneously fostered a social climate that made it possible to acknowledge a diverse range of impairments, and for people to identify themselves, or others, as invalids.[4]

Indeed, as David Turner and Daniel Blackie assert, 'disability was central to the Industrial Revolution ... Disabled people ... contributed to Britain's industrial development, while disability in turn shaped responses to industrialisation'.[5] Jose Harris notes how, by the late-Victorian and Edwardian periods, 'the immensely varied, contradictory, fissiparous quality of many movements, values, and institutions ... the riotous pluralism of human experience [were] embracing government, religion, work, family, moral attitudes, popular culture, and sexual relations'.[6] Such themes constitute a kaleidoscope of tensions and dynamics that exercised many comfortable minds, often conservative in outlook and therefore nervous of change and of aberration. It followed that some of their number were motivated to advance intervention in the lives of people with a diverse range of impairing circumstances. They often did this by marginalising them, moulding them, controlling them, segregating them and by confining them in the names of progress, rationalism, compassion and charity. Thus, a feature of the nineteenth century was the rise and the maturing of residential institutions for certain categories of disabled people. This resulted, for example, in people with mental impairments and afflictions being placed in asylums, or children and young people with sensory impairments being admitted to 'training' establishments.

By the Victorian period, mental asylums had become established features in the landscape, usually occupying rural locations. Onset of mental impairment had no respect of societal pedigree, but there were divergent responses as regards social class, gender and marital status. Within asylums, classification divided inmates between curable and incurable, tranquil and furious, rich and poor, men and women, young and old. Indeed, the Victorian period saw the rise of a range of institutions: physically, in stunning grandeur as elaborate edifices of stone and mortar; but also organisationally, as religiously and philanthropically motivated fraternities and societies. These were particularly inspired by the values of the increasingly influential middle classes, while they also solicited endorsement and patronage from the landed and aristocratic elites.[7]

The industrialists, manufacturers, traders, professionals, etc., who formed the upper strata of the rising middle classes, strove to emulate the landed classes by assuming guiding roles in civic society, a society that in the nineteenth century was increasingly bound by regulatory and legislative intervention and where formal philanthropic activity was a way of channelling elite energy. Business entrepreneurs maximised the financial returns on their capital through the labour of working-class men and women who toiled long hours, often in debilitating conditions that were compounded by overcrowded and unhealthy housing provision. It was therefore ironic that these elites were driven to founding and supporting societies and institutions to aid the victims of grinding hardship and of disabling conditions that were frequently the outcome of the desperate poverty that their business entrepreneurship played a part in creating. At the end of Victoria's reign, when Seebohm Rowntree published his social survey of York, he found that 'An analysis of the persons in the city who are below the "primary" poverty line shows that more than one half of these are members of families whose main wage-earner is in work but in receipt of insufficient wages.'[8]

As Sarah Rose has shown, expectations of ability to work often relegated disabled people to poverty and second-class citizenship.[9] Indeed, even as multiple definitions of disability operated during Britain's Industrial Revolution, disability was 'often associated with … a general incapacity for *any* kind of work', even as industry (e.g. coal mining) adopted occupational definitions of disability: one's capacity to work mattered more than inability to work.[10] The latter nineteenth century was a period marked by, in the words of Colin Barnes, 'A mixture of religious altruism and conscience, this spirit of Victorian patronage …'.[11] Religious altruism had a particularly motivating tenor in welfare provision, which, Stephen Yeo has noted, 'was an area in which churches and chapels were especially interested'.[12] Writing of the late-Victorian and Edwardian eras, Yeo continues, 'Such interest was regarded by many members of churches or chapels as automatically accompanying their religion as an especially religious province … total unconcern would have been unthinkable to many religious activists at this time.'[13] Religiosity, philanthropy and Victorian values of godliness, charity, sobriety and rational behaviour, hard work and desire for self-improvement, were inextricably intertwined.[14] Indeed, the elites were adept at marshalling the support of lower strata of society to embrace their values as their own. It formed part of a relentless process that is highlighted by Callum Brown:

> The great invention of evangelicalism was the voluntary organisation. It turned the elite organisation of eighteenth-century charity into the backbone of urban-industrial society, providing spiritual, educational, recreational, evangelising and moralising opportunities for the whole population ... The voluntary organisation took over the regulation of the people's habits from the established-church parish-state of the early modern period.[15]

The gestures of philanthropic industrialists and manufacturers, merchants, professionals and clergy were often driven by their own perceptions of acceptable lower-order work ethic and social responsibility, which they sought to generate among the working classes while also being motivated by their own interpretations of rational, religious and moral behaviour.[16] By the end of the Victorian period, elite altruism directed at social reform still involved marshalling working-class voluntary action, and created a two-pronged attack 'often called "service" when done by the rich, and "initiative" or "independence" when taken by the poor'.[17] Despite, for example, the widening of the political franchise for males, direction continued to emanate from above, and some of the top-down, well-meaning but value-laden actions by elites, for whom institutions and organisations that aimed at alleviating the effects of a range of disabling conditions had an enduring appeal, are demonstrated by our contributors in Parts I and II, on 'Attitudes' and 'Interventions'.

Queen Victoria's death in 1901 heralded the Edwardian era, in which there were some ideological changes in approaches to the support of those in need – such as children, the elderly, the sick, people whose circumstances might have been caused or aggravated by impairment or who were at risk of eventually becoming disabled. This occurred under legislation and actions dubbed the 'Liberal welfare reforms', but which some commentators have suggested were also spurred by early Labour Party electoral successes and pressure, rather than purely the pro-active initiative of a Liberal Party that drew its support from the middle classes and from skilled working-class voters who aspired to, and embraced, middle-class values. James Hay, for example, has noted 'that political pressure from the working class was one of the main reasons for the origins of social reform', and that 'both the Labour Party and the Trades Union Congress had extensive social reform programmes by the early 1900s'.[18]

However, despite the growth in state patronage of social welfare, introduced even as the onset of the Great War was anticipated, Victorian values and practices were to demonstrate considerable durability, casting a long and influential shadow across the twentieth century and beyond. The 1960s have been highlighted as the decade when 'Victorianism' underwent serious decline, the period that 'witnessed the decisive eclipse of "Victorian values"', but, as Ian Jones suggests in his study of religious change in Birmingham in the period after the Second World War, this is a simplistic judgement that is open to many challenges.[19] For example, Sue Wheatcroft notes that, in the post-war years of state intervention and welfare, 'many responsibilities previously met by the various voluntary societies' – which we recognise as being heavily embedded in the Victorian era – did not become obsolescent; rather, 'the role of charities changed, but in many ways they remained just as essential'.[20]

An advocate of the need for society to re-embrace Victorian values was Margaret Thatcher, Tory prime minister from 1979 to 1990, who equated the Victorian ethos as being 'entrepreneurial spirit, frugality and the authority of the family, all of them rooted in individual responsibility'.[21] Her espousal of Victorian values was cemented in a 1983 television interview when she revelled in the interviewer's suggestion that 'Victorian values' were what she stood for. Highlighting the likes of 'voluntary schools, [and] hospitals endowed by benefactors', she declared that 'as our people prospered, so they used their independence and initiative to prosper others, not compulsion by the State'.[22] Thatcher therefore had no hesitation in challenging the role of the wide-ranging welfare reforms that resulted from the Beveridge Report of 1942. Aspects of the continuity of the Victorian ethos in the face of change and modernity are showcased in the final section of this volume, 'Legacies'.[23]

Since the start of the twenty-first century, the number of different perceptions and understandings of what the term 'disability' represents have multiplied and caused significant argument and debate, 'disability' being both a relational and a value-laden concept.[24] The two dominant models of disability to prevail from the late twentieth century have been the medical model, stemming from clinical and scientific breakthroughs, notably from the nineteenth century, and the social model that defines disability as arising from societal attitudes and responses to impairment rather than from impairment itself. Advocates of the medical model have tended to posit disability as a 'problem' that needs to be 'fixed', with medical science playing the role of the knight in shining armour that will come to the rescue and banish disability. The social model argues that societal and political attitudes are the real problem, rather than the presence of a physiological impairment; but more recently there has been some compromise and overlap between these two models. Other models have also been recognised – such as the Expert or Professional model, the Tragedy or Charity model, the Moral model, the Legitimacy model, the Empowering model, the Economic model, the Market/Consumerist model and the Spectrum model – all aiming to appreciate the various lived experiences of disability.[25]

Within this 'new disability history', everybody's needs, aspirations and experiences are personal to them and dogmatic stances have consequently softened.[26] New perspectives argue away from a 'same, not different' perspective to a cultural interpretation that identifies 'same *and* different'.[27] Hughes and Paterson highlight that aspiration for a more inclusive, understanding and tolerant world, which does away with 'disability', and the lived reality of 'impairment', are not polar opposites and that we should acknowledge that 'disabled people experience impairment, as well as disability'.[28] Furthermore, as Burch and Rembis argue, '[d]isability is ubiquitous, yet it is also irreducible. Lived experiences of disability defy universalised or essentialised interpretations … there are many different ways to think about disability and disabled people.'[29] While several contributors to this volume are influenced by the social model, the editors do not take a dogmatic stance, enabling the collection to encompass medical perspectives, social arguments, cultural influences and the blurred and complex space between frameworks.

The collection has three contributions that explore aspects of hearing loss, notwithstanding debates surrounding whether deafness is a disability.[30] Many deaf people share negative perceptions of their situation, would prefer not to be deaf and share widely held outside perspectives that they are disabled as a consequence of their deafness.[31] However, this view is often not shared by people born deaf or losing their hearing at an early age; consequently, they feel no sense of loss and choose instead to celebrate their Deaf identity through their membership of a unique community and culture at the heart of which is sign language.[32] Yet, in both practical and legislative terms, deafness has been, and remains, explicitly classified as a disability. From 1861 until well into the twentieth century, the decennial censuses have recorded being 'deaf and dumb' in pathological terms, while definitions of disability within the 1948 National Assistance Act and the 1995 Disability Discrimination Act specifically cite deafness as a disabling condition. Deafness is not explicit in the 2010 Equality Act, but sensory impairment is included in guidance on determination of disability.[33]

Just as Claire Jones's collection of essays on the history of the commodification of prosthetic devices successfully combines those designed as substitute limbs alongside appliances created to aid recovery of hearing in the commercialisation of enabling accessories, this volume embraces hearing loss alongside essays that explore sight loss and mental and physical impairment.[34] The volume therefore concurs with the contemporary argument, advanced by Burch and Kafer, of 'the need for deaf/disability alliances'.[35] To showcase these alliances, but also to demonstrate the diversity of experiences and approaches within a particular strand of impairment, this collection takes deafness and hearing loss to highlight how one strand of impairment can occupy a broad landscape – and this model can, of course, be applied in other areas. So, in Part I, Attitudes, we see the conduct of deaf 'elite' personalities on the imperial stage (Chapter 2); in Part II, Interventions, we witness the medicalisation of deafness in clinics and hospitals (Chapter 4), and the linkages made between hearing impairment and childhood language development (Chapter 6); while in Part III, Legacies, Chapter 10 assesses the roots of continuing government policy mind-sets towards deafness as a disability. All these chapters use hearing loss to illustrate just some of the variety that can be identified under the broad umbrella terms of 'disability' and 'impairment'.

In this, and in other ways, *Disability and the Victorians* is intentionally varied. Just as the Victorian period was not just an era in time neatly bracketed between 1837 and 1901, the attitudes and outlooks generated reached beyond the British Isles – to Empire (Victoria became 'Empress of India' in 1886) and to the wider world. Medical, philanthropic, political and other elites engaged across frontiers through correspondence and investigative tours as they developed their individual philosophies, institutions and goals. Global journeys required considerable time to undertake, yet tours to Europe, North America and further afield were made by the likes of institution superintendents and philanthropic heavyweights in order to garner information on the perspectives and methods of their foreign counterparts and to exchange ideas. Thus, the Victorian reach and interface travelled far and wide – as two of our contributors, Esme Cleall and Caroline Lieffers, demonstrate in Chapters 2 and 7.

We argue that the Victorian gaze and influence endured long after the conclusion of a rigidly defined Victorian era. Victorian 'values' reverberated across the Edwardian period, through two world wars and into the decades of the British welfare state from its creation in 1948. We present examples of this in Part III by treading the established historical path of considering continuity and change. By the beginning of the twentieth century, the use of large institutions of various forms of confinement was increasingly challenged, but they were by then such established features of permanency on the landscape, representing considerable investment and serving as statements of philanthropic and civic largesse, that their continued role, irrespective of how inappropriate detractors might consider them to be, was simply because they 'already exist'.[36] Many of these buildings eventually underwent a process of identity change, such as becoming hospitals from 1948, or undergoing decommissioning from the 1980s. Examples still dot the landscape, some remaining in use as places of healthcare, some as majestic ruins, while some have been rehabilitated into new uses such as upmarket residential apartment complexes or educational establishments.

The diverse mix of contributions that comprises *Disability and the Victorians* comes from scholars whose writing demonstrates the profound impact that Victorian thinking and action had on shaping societal perceptions of physical, sensory and mental impairment and in establishing social responses, not only in Britain but also on the wider world stage. As stated earlier, the chapters primarily take a historical perspective, but contributions are included that demonstrate the growing and complementary overlap between 'pure' history and, for example, literary studies' use of disability as a genre, as demonstrated by Deborah Fratz in Chapter 3. Therefore, because of the heterogeneous nature of Victorian responses to impairment, the volume includes contributions that range from representations of impairment and disability in popular fiction, childhood language development and lived experiences of people in confinement, through to the disabling nature of alcohol dependency and abuse. These sit alongside more recognisable approaches on care provision, as showcased in chapters on deafness, blindness, prosthetics and medical care. Collectively, the chapters illustrate multifaceted understanding of the driving forces behind outsider intervention and insider experience in a way not usually found in disability history compendiums.

Overall, the volume does not set out to pursue the likes of Marxist or feminist perspectives. However, readers will find that individual contributors highlight experiences and approaches directed to varying degrees by, for example, gender (Chapters 5 and 7), social class (Chapters 1, 4, 5, 7, 10), work (Chapters 5 and 7) and ethnicity (Chapter 2). In marshalling the chapters under our three broad categories of Attitudes, Interventions and Legacies, we stress that these are not intended to be mutually exclusive, and we hope that the reader will find recurring themes and issues evident throughout the book.

Part I: Attitudes

Our collection begins with an examination of ways in which a variety of impairments were viewed by our Victorian forebears. These chapters explore the motivations that underpinned Victorian responses to people needing, and meriting, help and support – often with the objective of turning people experiencing debilitating infirmity or impairment into active and contributing members of society. This section investigates ways in which elites, in pursuit of their agendas of improvement, drove, for example, the establishment of voluntary hospitals in Scotland. It demonstrates how notions of physical and moral reform were exported across the British Empire. And it shows how perceptions of disability and chronic illness became a literary trope in the genre of 'Realism', revealing the depth of the perspectives of the comfortable classes and leading to their enrichment of all aspects of the Victorian psyche.

Amy Farnbach Pearson (Chapter 1) opens Part I by exploring the values and motivations of charitably funded voluntary hospitals, established by middle-class elites as places of cure for people experiencing chronic illness or impairment. Focusing on Glasgow Royal Infirmary (GRI) and the Royal Infirmary of Edinburgh (RIE), she shows how Scotland was an influential location in developing and disseminating the medical developments of the Victorian era, underpinned by middle-class ideals of restoring the deserving able-bodied from temporary illness or impairment to productive industry that energised the voluntary hospitals. This perspective of worthiness enacted at GRI and RIE reflected hardening societal attitudes towards the working classes, a tendency that increased during the nineteenth century among the middle classes throughout the British Isles. However, early and mid-Victorian reformers ultimately became disillusioned as they sensed failure in their efforts to restore significant numbers of individuals with impairments to able-bodiedness.

The Victorian period was the era during which the British Empire reached the zenith of its power and influence. The Empire presented opportunity to a wide spectrum of entrepreneurs, government administrators, military personnel, missionaries, adventurers, emigrants and refugees from the mother country. By exploring the life histories of three deaf educators and social reformers, Esme Cleall (Chapter 2) examines how these disabled white Britons fitted into the imperial matrix. John Kitto (1804–54), George Tait (1828–1904) and Jane Groom (1839–1918) can all, in some ways, be said to have lived imperial lives and to have adopted imperial attitudes to their surroundings. Cleall notes that, as disabled/deaf 'others', these were individuals who might be expected to empathise with the dispossessed indigenous peoples of colonised lands in their shared subjugation. However, she argues that they were all 'guilty' to some extent of embracing the imperialist project and of identifying with the coloniser rather than with the dispossessed and marginalised 'other'.

Disability history has a close association with aspects of literary studies, with numerous Victorian novelists perhaps being influenced, and inspired, by their personal experiences of impairing conditions. Among their ranks are Mary Elizabeth Braddon (1835–1915), Charlotte Brontë (1816–55), Wilkie Collins (1824–89), Dinah Craik (1826–87), Charles Dickens (1812–70), Elizabeth Gaskell (1810–65), Thomas Hardy (1840–1928), Robert Louis Stevenson (1850–94), Bram Stoker (1847–1912) and Charlotte Yonge (1823–1901). Deborah Fratz's (Chapter 3) exploration of representations of impairment and disability in the 'Literary Realism' writings of George Eliot (1819–90) and Harriet Martineau (1802–76) concludes Part I. Key to this genre are personal experience and social observation, which, Fratz argues, placed these authors and their literary methodology in a unique position to develop their characters' familiarity with living with impairment. Observation, by the characters and their creators, pinpoints perceptions within wider Victorian society and prevailing social interaction. The characters and their authors thus serve to perpetuate Victorian attitudes towards disabled people, not only for their contemporaneous readers, but for those who continue to read these classic titles today.

Part II: Interventions

Defining and confronting disability has taken various forms through the course of history; the Victorian period witnessed increased institutionalisation of people with impairments, marking their removal from mainstream society for periods ranging from short-term to life-long duration. The aim and aspiration of social reformers was disabled people's eventual return to the outside world as 'whole' beings, although for some this was neither achieved nor achievable. Places entrusted with objectives of rehabilitation, restoration to health and usefulness, and grooming for societal integration, included schools, hospitals, institutions, asylums, workhouses and poorhouses, sheltered workshops and centres of therapy and convalescence. In order to determine who was eligible to 'benefit' from such innovations, legislation, rules and tests were introduced to hone criteria by which people with wide-ranging and complex features of disablement could be categorised and directed towards different forms of intervention.

Interventions, the overriding theme of the chapters by Virdi (Chapter 4), Woiak (Chapter 5) and Hellal and Lorch (Chapter 6), therefore forms our second group of contributions, their themes providing insight to the inevitable outcome of Attitudes. Part II concludes with an alternative response from Lieffers (Chapter 7), which recognises that there were also people with disabilities who were not subjected to institutional regimes. The chapter highlights 'passing' as one strategy of confronting disablement within the context of the public sphere, and persuasively argues a consumer model of disability experience.[37]

Jaipreet Virdi begins the theme of Interventions by considering practical, medical and technological responses to deafness. It was during the nineteenth century that specialist hospitals emerged, but medical specialisation was often ridiculed by general clinicians who took pride in having training and expertise that they felt equipped them to direct their skills to any kind of medical challenge. In their view, specialisation, from paediatrics to psychiatry, was the refuge of colleagues who lacked their own wide-ranging abilities and versatility. In Chapter 4 Virdi outlines the arguments put forward by those opposed to specialisation. It was a contest that they were destined to lose. She demonstrates the shift towards a more medicalised construction of deafness by examining the evolution of London's Royal Dispensary for Diseases of the Ear (RDDE) and its approaches to the specialist treatment that it advocated. In due course, the RDDE became the Royal Ear Hospital, and Virdi charts the institution's progress and development from its foundation in the pre-Victorian early nineteenth century to the post-Victorian early twentieth century.

The debates surrounding what constitutes 'disability' and what are considered appropriate reactions to disabling conditions are highlighted poignantly, perhaps even controversially, in Joanne Woiak's examination in Chapter 5 of the historical background to psychiatric, eugenic and wider societal responses to inebriation. Discourses and policies that connected the concepts of alcoholism and degeneration were prominent targets around which disability was constructed in the Victorian and Edwardian eras. Woiak emphasises the roles that gender and social class played in eliciting contradictory responses – responses that demonstrated either compassion or prejudice towards the debilitating effects of alcohol addiction. She considers the competing arguments of the teetotal movement, social Darwinists and eugenicists, alongside the emerging medical disciplines of psychiatry and public health, to create a complex narrative about whether alcoholism should have been universally recognised as a disability during the Victorian period, and if Victorian attitudes continue to impact on contemporary thinking and discourses on alcohol dependency.

Medical surveillance in the interest of expanding clinical knowledge provides the focus for Paula Hellal and Marjorie Lorch's chapter on the linkage between perceptions of sensory impairment, in this case the ability to hear and to articulate, and learning development. The authors explore Victorian attitudes to childhood disability by focusing on how physicians attempted to describe and explain these newly identified developmental disorders of language. Focusing primarily on childhood aphasia, they highlight the haphazard ways in which the medical profession made breakthroughs to achieve greater understanding of the condition. This required abandonment of early ideas, which had often been without empirical foundation, in order to embrace fresh perspectives and understanding and to reappraise the long-held and dubious linkage made between deafness and 'dumbness'. Hellal and Lorch outline how research into childhood health conditions and disabilities was initially largely driven by individual interest and became more systematic only once hospitals brought together a large number of people, enabling greater understanding of various physiological conditions so as to benefit from medical collaboration.

There were, of course, people with disabilities who played active roles within able-bodied society, but life with a physical or sensory impairment in the public sphere took on many manifestations. Integration within mainstream society might mean endeavouring to mask an impairment so as to avoid stereotyping or being on the receiving end of false assumptions by people encountered during daily life. Therefore, adopting a strategy of hiding an impairment – or 'passing' as able-bodied – motivated the likes of the insertion of a false eye or employing a range of other devices to make invisible an absent, malformed or damaged body part or function.

'Passing' was an objective of the prosthetic limb developed by Benjamin Franklin Palmer, and which is investigated by Caroline Lieffers in Chapter 7. Palmer was adept at marketing the benefits of his prosthetic devices in both practical and aesthetic terms by aligning his inventions with medical progress. He adhered to what Lieffers identifies as a medical-consumerist model where Palmer's prosthesis became a sought-after accessory based on medical innovation and modernity. Thus he capitalised on testimonials from satisfied customers: the prosthesis, wearers suggested, was able to merge with the body, making them 'whole' again, physically and psychologically; and it facilitated masculine ideals of sociability, labour and business success. For the wearer, it enabled life to be conducted as 'normal'. International marketing of Palmer's invention created a following for a device that was 'conspicuously inconspicuous'. Palmer's successful global outreach demonstrated that Victorian values and ideals were not limited to Britain and its empire; his invention originated at a local level in the 'new world', but eventually extended its appeal and success throughout the United States, and across the Atlantic to the 'old world'.

Part III: Legacies

Our final section highlights examples of how the shadow cast by our Victorian forebears has been a long one. In Chapter 8 Iain Hutchison traces the ways in which the treatment of chronically ill and disabled children evolved in late nineteenth-century Scotland and how those Victorian approaches and principles continued to evolve in the early decades of the twentieth century. Direct experience of the consequences of such institutional attitudes is explored in Chapter 9 through Fred Reid's very personal narration and analysis of his adolescent life and development in a residential blind school where surveillance, often guided by a Victorian mind-set, was the order of the day. Martin Atherton concludes the volume with his examination, in Chapter 10, of how government policy and practice directed at deaf and hearing-impaired people, from the nineteenth century through to the early twenty-first century, has often replicated, rather than challenged, the thinking that was prevalent in the Victorian period.

The ambiguous nature of the boundary between ill health and disability becomes apparent in Iain Hutchison's chapter on the experience of feeble, frail, ill and impaired children in Glasgow. In opening Part III of this collection, Hutchison provides a longitudinal review of the interrelationship between Glasgow's Royal Hospital for Sick Children (RHSC), its use of a network of 'cottages' to aid post-treatment recovery, and East Park Home for Infirm Children, an institution created to aid children with a range of disabling conditions. He illustrates how the shortcomings of compulsory education from 1872, and the belated arrival of a children's hospital in 1883, precipitated a new approach to children with serious physical impairments, and traces continuity of the Victorian ethos when the children's hospital, and charity-run convalescence homes, evolved rather than transformed in the aftermath of the Great War. From the inter-war period, a close relationship developed between the RHSC and East Park Home, where residential and education facilities were provided for children with a broad and changing spectrum of impairing conditions, and which today continues to operate as an educational facility for children with disabilities.

Fred Reid's story gives a very personal insight into the continuity of Victorian values and practices well into the immediate post-Second World War era. Using his 2006 novella, *The Panopticon*, which is based on his own lived experience of growing up in a residential blind home and school during the middle of the twentieth century, Reid argues that the paternal ethos of residential institutions for disabled people nonetheless resulted in intrusive surveillance. His particular focus is on how personal relationships between pupils were regulated and impeded, and on the ways in which transgressions of the strict moral code of the institution were punished. While acknowledging the benefits that communal living with contemporaries could provide, he explains how residential schools failed to prepare teenagers for the emotional, romantic and sexual challenges of adolescence and adult life.

Rather than taking a linear approach from the Victorian era to modern times to evaluate continuity or change in categorising people with disabilities and, in particular, people with hearing loss, in Chapter 10 Martin Atherton examines the mind-sets that frame twentieth- and early twenty-first-century UK government policy. He argues that thinking which continues to marginalise deaf people from opportunities for meaningful employment, can be traced to roots in the Poor Law legislation for England and Wales of 1834. Although the last vestiges of the Poor Law were finally abolished by the creation of a welfare state in 1948, Atherton contends that, in practice, its ethos continues by excluding deaf and disabled people through placing emphasis on assumptions about what an individual might be unable to do, rather than on what they *can* do. He reveals how this results in low self-esteem and lack of self-belief – despite legislative trends aimed at creating a more equal and inclusive society.

Disability and the Victorians: Attitudes, interventions, legacies

Much has been written about disability, its construction and representation during the nineteenth century. There is a growing literature about the lived experience of impairing conditions during that time, and especially when it coincided with maturation of manufacturing and industry, urbanisation, medical investigation and discovery, political realignment as the electoral franchise widened, and imperial expansion on the back of demographic change and the global consolidation of military power. This period has become associated with Victorianism, not least because of the longevity of Queen Victoria's reign. The people who lived during the years between 1837 and 1901, and especially those who prospered, became The Victorians. They left their imprint, but people with a kaleidoscopic array of impairments were often the ones on whom that imprint left an enduring impression.

The ten chapters presented in *Disability and the Victorians* do not pretend to offer a comprehensive overview of how impairment was experienced, perceived or controlled during and beyond the Victorian decades, but aim to provide both a small sample of the variability of disability presentation and experience, and a taste of how the ethos that was spawned during the Victorian period was so powerful that it reverberated through the decades that followed. The historian's work is never done, and so it is with *Disability and the Victorians*. The contributions to this volume are intended to stimulate the reader, but also to generate debate and spur further research, to encourage exposition of the diversity of the Victorian dynamic and its reverberations across space and time. If our authors can achieve a little of that as an agenda, our pens can perhaps rest for just a short time before we again embark on the endless task of exploring disability in historical context, not just in the Victorian era but across the centuries – and across continents.

Notes

1 A. Borsay, *Disability and Social Policy in Britain since 1750* (Basingstoke: Palgrave Macmillan, 2005); A. Borsay (ed.), *Medicine in Wales, c. 1800–2000: Public Service or Private Commodity?* (Cardiff: University of Wales Press, 2003); V. Crossman, *Poverty and the Poor Law in Ireland, 1850–1914* (Liverpool: Liverpool University Press, 2013); L. H. Lees, *The Solidarities of Strangers: The English Poor Laws and the People, 1700–1948* (Cambridge: Cambridge University Press, 1998); I. Levitt, *Poverty and Welfare in Scotland, 1890–1948* (Edinburgh: Edinburgh University Press, 1988); D. S. Lucey, *The End of the Irish Poor Law: Welfare and Healthcare Reform in Revolutionary Ireland* (Manchester: Manchester University Press, 2015);

R. Mitchison, *The Old Poor Law in Scotland: the Experience of Poverty, 1574–1845* (Edinburgh: Edinburgh University Press, 2000).

2   Borsay, *Disability and Social Policy.*

3   S. King, *Poverty and Welfare in England: 1700–1850* (Manchester: Manchester University, 2000); Lees, *The Solidarity of Strangers*; L. Charlesworth, *Welfare's Forgotten Past: A Socio-Legal History of the Poor Law* (London: Routledge-Cavendish, 2012).

4   M. H. Frawley, *Invalidism and Identity in Nineteenth-century Britain* (Chicago, IL: University of Chicago Press, 2004).

5   D. M. Turner and D. Blackie, *Disability in the Industrial Revolution: Physical Impairment in British Coalmining, 1780–1880* (Manchester: Manchester University Press, 2018), p. 2.

6   J. Harris, *Private Lives, Public Spirit: Britain 1870–1914* (London: Penguin, 1994), p. 2.

7   For discussion on mental asylum development, see, for example, A. Scull, *Museums of Madness: The Social Organization of Insanity in Nineteenth-Century England* (London: Allen Lane, 1979); J. Melling and B. Forsythe (eds), *Insanity, Institutions and Society, 1800–1914* (London: CRC Press, 2014); R. Porter, *A Social History of Madness: Stories of the Insane* (London: Phoenix Giants, 1996); M. Foucault, *Madness and Civilization: A History of Insanity in the Age of Reason* (London: Routledge, 2001).

8   B. S. Rowntree, *Poverty: A Study of Town Life* ([London: Macmillan, 1901], Bristol: Policy Press, 2000), p. 114.

9   S. F. Rose, *No Right to Be Idle: The Invention of Disability, 1840s–1930s* (Durham, NC: University of North Carolina Press, 2017). See also M. O'Cathain, '"Blind, but not to the hard facts of life": the blind workers' struggle in Derry, 1928–1940', *Radical History Review*, 94 (2006), 9–21.

10 D. Blackie, 'Disability and work during the Industrial Revolution in Britain', in M. Rembis, C. Kudlick, and K. E. Nielsen (eds), *The Oxford Handbook of Disability History* (Oxford: Oxford University Press, 2018), pp. 177–93; 185–6.

11 C. Barnes, *Disabled People in Britain and Discrimination* (London: Hurst, 1991), p. 16.

12 S. Yeo, *Religion and Voluntary Organisations in Crisis* (London: Croom Helm, 1976), p. 57.

13 *Ibid.*

14 T. C. Smout (ed.), *Proceedings of the British Academy: Victorian Values*, p. 78 (1992).

15 C. G. Brown, *The Death of Christian Britain* (London: Routledge, 2001), p. 45.

16 G. Himmelfarb, 'The age of philanthropy', *The Wilson Quarterly*, 21:2 (1997), 48–55; F. Prochaska, *Christianity and Social Service in Modern Britain: The Disinherited Spirit* (Oxford: Oxford University Press, 2006).

17 Yeo, *Religion and Voluntary Organisations*, p. 220.

18 J. R. Hay, *The Origins of the Liberal Welfare Reforms, 1906–14*, 2nd edn (Basingstoke: Macmillan, 1983), pp. 25–7.

19 I. Jones, *The Local Church and Generational Change in Birmingham, 1945–2000* (Woodbridge: Boydell Press, 2012), p. 155.

20 S. Wheatcroft, *Worth Saving: Disabled Children during the Second World War* (Manchester: Manchester University Press, 2013), p. 171.

21 P. Jenkins, *Mrs Thatcher's Revolution: The Ending of the Socialist Era* (Cambridge, MA: Harvard University Press, 1988), p. 67.

22 C. Moore, *Margaret Thatcher: The Authorized Biography*, vol. II (London: Allen Lane, 2015), pp. 8–9.

23 W. Beveridge, *Social Insurance and Allied Services* (London: War Cabinet, 1942).

24 T. Shakespeare, 'The social model of disability', in L. Davis (ed.), *The Disability Studies Reader* (London: Taylor and Francis, 2016), pp. 195–203; C. Barnes and G. Mercer (eds), *Exploring Disability* (Cambridge: Polity Press, 2010); L. Barton, C. Barnes and M. Oliver, *Disability Studies Today* (Cambridge: Polity Press, 2002); I. Hutchison, *A History of Disability in Nineteenth-Century Scotland* (Lewiston: Mellen, 2007), pp. 3–8; D. M. Turner, 'Introduction: approaching anomalous bodies', in D. M. Turner and K. Stagg (eds), *Social Histories of Disability and Deformity* (New York, NY: Routledge, 2006), p. 2.

25 www.disabled-world.com/definitions/disability-models.php, accessed 10 January 2019.

26 P. K. Longmore and L. Umansky, 'Disability history: from the margins to the mainstream', in P. K. Longmore and K. Umansky (eds), *The New Disability History: American Perspectives* (New York, NY and London: New York University Press, 2001), pp. 1–29.

27 P. Devlieger, F. Rusch and D. Pieffer (eds), *Rethinking Disability: The Emergence of New Definitions, Concepts and Communities* (Antwerp: Garant, 2003), p. 9.

28 B. Hughes and K. Paterson, 'The social model of disability and the disappearing body: towards a sociology of impairment', *Disability & Society*, 12:3 (1997), 334.

29 S. Burch and M. Rembis, 'Re-membering the past: reflections on disability histories', in S. Burch and M. Rembis (eds), *Disability Histories* (Urbana, Chicago, IL: University of Illinois Press, 2014), p. 1.

30 See, for example, M. Corker, *Deaf and Disabled or Deafness Disabled?* (Buckingham: Open University Press, 1998); V. Finkelstein, 'We are not disabled, you are', in S. Gregory and G. M. Hartley (eds), *Constructing Deafness* (London: Pinter Publishers, 1991), pp. 265–71; H. Lane, 'Do deaf people have a disability?', address at the Federation of Deaf People conference, Blackburn, 7 November 1998.

31 P. Higgins, *Outsiders in a Hearing World* (London: Sage, 1980); J. Ballantyne and J. A. M. Martin, *Deafness* (Edinburgh: Livingstone, 1984); D. Wright, *Deafness: A Personal Account* (London: Allen Lane, 1969).

32 J. Harris, *The Cultural Meaning of Deafness* (Aldershot: Avebury, 1995); B. Grant, *The Deaf Advance* (Edinburgh: Pentland, 1990); R. Lee (ed.), *Deaf Liberation* (London: National Union of the Deaf, 1992); G. Taylor and J. Bishop (eds), *Being Deaf: The Experience of Deafness* (London: Pinter Publishers, 1991); C. Padden, 'The deaf community and deaf culture', in Gregory and Hartley (eds), *Constructing Deafness* (London: Pinter Publishers, 1991), pp. 40–5, at p. 44. For more on the formation of deaf/hearing-impaired communities, see R. A. R. Edwards, *Words Made Flesh:*

Nineteenth-CENTURY Deaf Education and the Growth of Deaf Culture (New York, NY: New York University Press, 2012); J. Esmail, *Reading Victorian Deafness: Signs and Sounds in Victorian Literature and Culture* (Ohio, OH: Ohio University Press, 2013); G. Gooday and K. Sayer, *Managing the Experience of Hearing Loss in Britain, 1830–1930* (London and New York, NY: Palgrave Macmillan, 2017).

33 *Equality Act 2010: Guidance* (London: Her Majesty's Stationery Office, 2010), p. 8.

34 C. Jones (ed.), *Rethinking Modern Prosthetics in Anglo-American Commodity Cultures, 1820–1939* (Manchester: Manchester University Press, 2017).

35 S. Burch and A. Kafer (eds), *Deaf and Disability Studies: Interdisciplinary Perspectives* (Washington, DC: Gallaudet University Press, 2010), p. xvii.

36 J. K. Love, *The Deaf Child: A Manual for Teachers and School Doctors* (Bristol: John Wright, 1911), p. 134.

37 J. A. Brune and D. J. Wilson, 'Introduction', in J. A. Brune and D. J. Wilson (eds), *Disability and Passing: Blurring in the Lines of Identity* (Philadelphia, PA: Temple University Press, 2013), p. 1.

Part I

ATTITUDES

I

RESTORATION TO USEFULNESS: VICTORIAN MIDDLE-CLASS ATTITUDES TOWARDS THE HEALTHCARE OF THE WORKING POOR

Amy W. Farnbach Pearson

Early and mid-Victorian social reformers were optimistic regarding the middle classes' ability to steer Britain towards a more prosperous future.[1] Social action, sanitary reforms and medical science could be deployed to improve the condition of the working classes and cure their ills.[2] However, the incurable, those whose disorders medical practitioners deemed refractory to treatment, presented a challenging barrier to this idealism and optimism.

In Victorian Britain, members of the working classes were more vulnerable than those of the middle and upper classes to physical impairment through industrial accidents, and to diseases such as tuberculosis, cholera, influenza and typhus due to crowded living conditions and privation.[3] At the same time, their treatment in voluntary hospitals depended upon their adherence to middle-class standards of behaviour, including industriousness. As many individuals with long-term illness or impairment were either unable to maintain manual jobs or were excluded from doing so, they risked social classification among the so-called 'idle poor' and could therefore be deemed unfit for treatment. As a result, health status and social status interacted recursively, forging a conceptual link between individuals with chronic illness or impairment and the increasingly marginalised working classes. The medical establishment's ineffective amelioration of the health risks facing the working classes intersected with middle-class preoccupations with working-class reform to render the 'cure' of impairment socially as well as medically significant, engendering social disability and the stigma of impairment.

This process will be investigated through case studies drawn from two major Scottish voluntary hospitals, Glasgow Royal Infirmary (GRI) and the Royal Infirmary of Edinburgh (RIE). Scotland was influential in developing and disseminating the medical developments of the Victorian era. For example, Scotland led the British Isles in adopting the new stethoscope,[4] which allowed practitioners to base diagnosis on the inference of internal pathology[5] rather than on the external examination favoured during the eighteenth century.[6] Scotland was also at the forefront of advancing infection control in hospitals under the influence of surgeons such as Joseph Lister (1827–1912) who advocated use of antiseptic measures in GRI and the RIE.[7]

Scotland further offered medical students accessible academic and practical training. Scottish medical education included pharmacology and surgery as well as clinical medicine.[8] GRI touted affordable tuition rates, boasting in 1835 that 'medical instruction ... got for seven guineas in Glasgow, would in London cost above fifty, and in Edinburgh nearly twenty pounds'.[9] Knowledge of Latin, a requirement for medical degrees throughout Europe, was somewhat de-emphasised in Glasgow and Edinburgh, such that individuals with only a 'shaky' grasp of the language preferred to receive medical training there.[10] As a result, medical education acquired at GRI, the RIE and elsewhere in Scotland, while well respected, was also accessible to those with a moderate income. This approach proved popular in Scotland and beyond, with three-quarters of Edinburgh graduates at the turn of the nineteenth century originating outside of Scotland, and half from beyond the British Isles.[11]

Because of its more moderate cost and less lofty admission requirements, as well as the blurring, from the mid-seventeenth century, of the distinctions among apothecaries, surgeons and physicians, medical training in Scotland created a more cohesive and egalitarian practitioner workforce than elsewhere in Britain.[12] The diversity of the economic status of Scottish practitioners is evident from the prevalence in Scotland of medical shop-keeping – an important activity for doctors who found themselves unable to live off their practice consulting fees alone, and so set themselves up as pharmacists to supplement their income.[13] Nonetheless, qualification as a physician required a university degree in Scotland as elsewhere in the United Kingdom, limiting the profession on which this chapter focuses to individuals of at least middle-class education and economic status.

Both GRI and the RIE were founded in the eighteenth century with the aim of providing comprehensive medical training to student practitioners and charitable medical care to the 'worthy poor', i.e. the working poor as opposed to the 'idle poor'. The managers of these hospitals held the treatment of the idle poor to be the responsibility of those individuals' home parishes and, following the 1845 Poor Law Amendment (Scotland) Act, increasingly relied upon rate-funded poorhouses to make hospital provision for paupers. The voluntary hospitals were supported through donations and subscriptions. Subscribers, which included employers, trade guilds, friendly societies, charitable organisations and patrons, paid an annual amount for the privilege of recommending patients to the infirmary. Except for the victims of accidents, prospective patients generally would not be granted admission to the infirmary without a ticket of recommendation from a subscriber. Voluntary hospitals such as GRI and the RIE were not generally patients' first choice for treatment. Those who could afford to pay preferred treatment at home, in physicians' or surgeons' consultation rooms, at apothecary shops or from lay practitioners. Hospitals, it was popularly believed, experimented on patients; following the 1832 Anatomy Act, poor patients and their families also feared post-mortem dissection.[14] For much of the nineteenth century, hospital treatment was sought only *in extremis.* Even so, GRI and the RIE each treated more than 4,000 patients annually in the period 1837 to 1901.[15]

The particular focus of this chapter is on patients impaired by chronic disease, most commonly tuberculosis (TB) and related diagnoses such as consumption and phthisis. Even today, TB is most prevalent among marginalised people; during the nineteenth century, it gained significance as a benchmark for the health of the social body in Great Britain and the Western world more broadly.[16] TB among working-class individuals was of particular concern during the latter half of the century, during which the middle classes increasingly exerted themselves in efforts to 'improve' the working classes, and at the turn of the century, when physical degeneration was increasingly invoked to explain their poorer health. While TB can affect the bones and joints, digestive system, genitourinary system and skin, the lungs were the most common site of tubercular disease recorded by medical staff in Victorian-era ward journals at GRI and the RIE. Because of this, and because practitioners in medical wards recorded more detailed case notes than did surgical practitioners, the patients discussed in this chapter are most commonly medical cases diagnosed with pulmonary tubercular disorders rather than surgical cases.

'A great number of maimed [persons] may be seen going about'[17]

Scottish medical practitioners embraced the new technologies and increasing knowledge about health and disease that marked the early nineteenth century. During this time, improved accessibility of post-mortem dissection afforded by the 1832 Anatomy Act, and increasing interest among practitioners regarding the manifestations and aetiology of disease, spurred the development of evidence-based medical practice.[18] While this generated optimism that more effective treatments must follow, the most prevalent threats to health – epidemics of diseases such as cholera and typhus, chronic disorders like TB, and permanent injury – remained formidable throughout the nineteenth century, particularly for the working classes.[19] Overcrowded housing, malnutrition, industrial hazards and exposure to infectious disease experienced by the working classes of the Victorian era led to greater prevalence of illness and physical impairment when compared to their wealthier contemporaries. Repeated contagion episodes during the early Victorian period made it clear to contemporary observers that morbidity and mortality from infectious disease were concentrated in poor, urban neighbourhoods, rendering these areas as targets for control efforts.[20]

Chronic disease also disproportionately affected the working classes. By the mid-nineteenth century, public health advocates recognised that TB was more common among low-income and otherwise marginalised groups.[21] TB authority and RIE physician John Hughes Bennett (1812–75) argued that the working classes were more susceptible due to inadequate nutrition.[22] For Bennett, consumption was not a disease of *able-bodied* [original emphasis] men ... whatever [their] privations', but, rather, of 'the young of foundling hospitals, factories and the poor and labouring classes'.[23] Indeed, by the twentieth century, authorities on the disease invoked a common aphorism: 'There are two kinds of consumption – that of the rich and that of the poor. The former is sometimes cured, the latter never.'[24]

Bennett's implicit exclusion of 'the poor and labouring classes' from the ranks of the 'able-bodied' is telling. Industrial hazards placed factory labourers at high risk of impairment, a circumstance described at length in 1844 by Frederick Engels (1820–95) in *The Condition of the Working-class in England*. Engels wrote of 'a peculiar deformity of the shoulder' and 'diseases of the knee-pan' resulting from work in spinning mills.[25] This was in addition to amputation accidents with the result that 'besides the deformed persons, a great number of maimed ones may be seen going about in Manchester; ... it is like living in the midst of an army just returned from a campaign.'[26] Therefore, by the early Victorian period, a critical concentration of disease, impairment and early death among the working classes was clear in the minds of medical practitioners and social reformers alike. Indeed, the 'condition of the masses' novels, as well as labour and sanitary reforms undertaken at this time, testify to the concern for the state of the working classes among the middle class more broadly.

'Restoration for a time to industry and usefulness'[27]

The physical state of productive labourers was a preoccupying concern of Victorian social thought owing to the importance of these workers' output to national – and middle-class – wealth.[28] Perhaps as a result, industriousness was salient among the traits marking working-class individuals as respectable through middle-class eyes. It follows that the working poor were considered the most appropriate recipients of charitable interventions, including voluntary hospitals like GRI and the RIE, to the exclusion of the so-called idle poor. Indeed, the importance of work was such that future prospects of good health, particularly the ability to work, in part determined individuals' status as 'worthy' of hospital charity.

From the turn of the nineteenth century, voluntary hospitals were advised to emphasise the treatment of curable cases. The Edinburgh-trained physician Thomas Percival (1740–1804), in his influential *Medical Ethics*, recommended that hospitals should prioritise the admission of those 'capable of speedy relief' so as to maximise the number of patients benefited by the hospital's resources.[29] In contrast, admissions of those 'under maladies incapable of relief' were to be avoided.[30] Failure to do so, Percival argued, would prevent the desirable 'quick change of objects' (i.e. patients) alluded to above, as well as place such patients at risk of hospital-borne infections, a source of 'almost certain death' for those staying in hospital for an extended period.[31] If hospital administrators felt regret at turning away incurable cases, Percival reassured them, 'The visitation of sickness is a wise and kind dispensation of Providence, intended to humble, to refine, and to meliorate the heart.'[32]

Into the Victorian era, the boards of management of GRI and the RIE continued to espouse Percival's recommendation to limit the admission of incurable patients, albeit with modification. At the turn of the nineteenth century, incurable patients might be summarily discharged. In 1798 Jean W, a phthisis patient at GRI, was dismissed as an 'improper' patient after eight days' stay, the medical staff noting that 'every complaint increases rapidly. Being no longer an object of medical treatment she is dismissed.'[33] During the Victorian period, patients classified as incurable by infirmary administrators and medical staff were given treatment, although this was commonly time limited. Mary D, admitted to the RIE with a dermatological disorder, showed little improvement over the course of thirty-seven days and was dismissed when the hospital became pressed for space, it being noted at her discharge that 'the beds were wanted very badly, she was dismissed today; not much relieved.'[34]

In principle, such admission and discharge policies privileging curable patients maximised these hospitals' use of limited funding, as recommended by Percival, by increasing patient turnover. At the RIE, the board of managers did face pressure from donors to reduce the average patient stay, so enabling the treatment of more patients annually.[35] To this end, the RIE advocated a sixty-day limit on hospital stays, although exceptions to this limit were routinely granted on the basis of medical expediency.[36] In 1844 the RIE board of managers sought to limit the increasing and expensive admission of incurable patients by reminding the medical staff that 'by careful selection of patients for admission, the expense may be properly diminished', specifying that 'the object of the establishment is to cure or relieve disease, and that patients neither capable of cure nor relief however much objects of pity ... ought not to be admitted here'.[37]

In practice, however, the focus on curable patients was refined by the importance of productive work in defining those 'worthy' of admission. As early as 1815, GRI touted its annual report, a document widely circulated in Glasgow to encourage donations to the hospital, as 'a catalogue of fellow creatures ... relieved from disease ... restored to health and strength – to useful occupation and domestic enjoyment', underscoring the hospital's role in reclaiming ill individuals from idleness.[38] The medical staff at the RIE, in replying to the board of managers' 1844 insistence that incurable patients be excluded, argued in part:

> that there are none which do not admit of some degree of relief; the only difference being, that some, although not curable, admit of relief for a considerable time, and even of restoration for a time to industry and usefulness, while others admit only of temporary alleviation of suffering.[39]

While the medical staff went on to advocate the admission of both types of patient, it is clear that their argument rested in part on the inclusion of 'restoration for a time to industry' alongside cure as a valid aim of the hospital.

In the same 1844 reply to the RIE board of managers' rejection of incurable patients, RIE medical practitioners countered the board's suggestion that incurable patients were 'fitted only for an Alms house' by asserting that existing poorhouse facilities at the time, prior to their expansion in response to the 1845 Poor Law Amendment (Scotland) Act, were 'on so limited a scale and generally so full, as to be unable to admit many such applicants'.[40] Instead, the medical staff argued, it was an obligation of the infirmary, as a voluntary charity, to relieve 'sufferings resulting from disease, even from such as are known to be incurable'.[41] It is important to note that poorhouses in Scotland had a role that was quite different from that of English workhouses. The New Poor Law (1845) in Scotland relieved only paupers who were 'disabled' from working, while England's New Poor Law (1834) included able-bodied paupers. Nonetheless, both before and after Scotland's Act, the RIE's board distinguished between individuals appropriate to receive relief at the infirmary versus the poorhouse, which, for the exclusively working-class patients of the RIE, was a distinction resting in part upon curability.

In contrast to boards of management, RIE medical staff in 1844 argued for the admission of individuals in need of skilled treatment as opposed to those cured easily, and espoused the value to medical education of admitting the full spectrum of diseases.[42] Detracting somewhat from the humanitarian tone of the argument as a whole, part of the educational value in treating incurable patients lay in the explicitly stated possibility that their dying in hospital could render their bodies available for dissection. The medical staff considered such post-mortems critical to medical training and medical science: 'let it be remembered', urged the medical staff, 'that a great part of the usefulness of the Hospital as a School of Medicine, consists in its exhibiting to the Students the fatal termination of diseases and the appearances in dissection.'[43]

Widespread post-mortem dissection of deceased poor patients in the United Kingdom and continental Europe was germinal to the nineteenth-century development of a self-consciously scientific medicine.[44] Wealthier private patients were also dissected in Scotland, but this was rarer and more dignified: the RIE's John Hughes Bennett informed students that organs could be examined *in situ*, and generally would be so in private post-mortems.[45] However, during his lecture dissections at the RIE – the subjects of which would have been bodies from the hospital – he would circulate body parts of interest among the students. The difference between rare private dissections and frequent dissections in the context of teaching hospitals lay in the necessity of poor bodies for training medical practitioners and advancing medical science. This emphasises that terminal patients were valued for their utility to the middle class, in much the same way as were able-bodied patients, who, it was hoped, would be returned to work after treatment.

A change in the distribution of hospital admissions occurred with the gradual implementation of the 1867 Public Health Act, which placed provision for fever patients in the sphere of municipal authorities and therefore increasingly away from voluntary hospitals. In Glasgow this process began with the opening, by Glasgow Town Council in 1870, of Belvedere Hospital for patients with infectious diseases. A decade later, the RIE's Committee of Contributors noted that fever patients tended to have longer confinements than either medical or surgical cases and questioned 'whether the expense of a Fever Hospital should continue to be undertaken by the Royal Infirmary, or placed under the provisions of the Public Health Act'.[46] The Committee had its way four years later when the RIE's fever hospital was acquired by Edinburgh Town Council and the Council assumed 'sole charge of all cases of infectious diseases occurring within the city'.[47]

By the turn of the twentieth century, medical staff at GRI began to record in patients' case notes, not only the duration of illness, but also how long the patient had been away from work, signalling an increased emphasis on the importance of labour status in identifying the worthy poor. When time out of work was not attributable to illness, the reasons were noted with distinct disapprobation. For example, Francis M, admitted in 1905 suffering from phthisis pulmonalis and alcoholism, was recorded by the medical staff as being 'a tinsmith by trade, but in the last three years has not done much, as his wife had a business and made sufficient for both'.[48]

To become unable to engage in productive labour was, for the Victorian working classes, to transition from 'worthy' to 'idle', potentially unfit for voluntary hospital aid, even 'useless'. Noyes attributes the suspicion with which those claiming illness or impairment without apparent somatic disorder came to be regarded as akin to industrialisation, which 'increased the value of health and the ability to work', consequently casting those unable to work as 'a burden on society'.[49] That this 'burden' was expected to be repaid by working-class individuals with illness and impairment through a return to productive labour, and, should they die in hospital, contribution to medical science and training through post-mortem dissection, resonates with sociologist Talcott Parsons' (1902–79) classic conception of illness as deviance, and underscores the recursive nexus between health status and social status.[50]

'Stunted, misshapen, and often loathsome objects'[51]

During the late-Victorian period illness among the lower orders became not just burdensome but loathsome in the eyes of middle-class reformers. If the cure of illness and impairment could restore individuals to respectability, it followed that incurable disorders and chronic disability were to be seen as discrediting to those affected. Indeed, both working-class status and poor health were considered to distance such individuals from the respectable middle classes as disreputable 'others'.[52] This conformed to the tendency of Victorian class relations to regard perceived class distinctions and health status as inhering in the working class-body owing to the contribution of productive work to middle-class norms of behaviour. The recursive relationship between the two, health status compromising one's ability to engage in appropriate labour, in turn marking one both economically and behaviourally as beyond the sphere of middle-class values, served to emphasise the 'otherness' of working-class individuals with illness and impairments and to stigmatise such conditions.

In Victorian Britain illness and impairment interacted with strong class distinctions to conflate the disvalued traits of members of the working classes with those of individuals with impairments. This occurred through the conflation of illness and impairment with idleness, as well as through prevailing social constructs of illness and health as matters of personal responsibility. For the Victorians, health was a quality to be actively maintained. Health or illness was the result of 'the sum of one's transactions with the environment', as well as careful self-control.[53] As the Edinburgh-trained physician J. Milner Fothergill (1841–88) explained in his lay health guide, *Maintenance of Health*, 'uncleanliness of the mind and body act and react, and perfect health of one is incompatible with an unhealthy state of the other'.[54]

Those at greater risk of disease had greater responsibility to engage in healthy behaviour, as with respect to the nineteenth-century concept of diathesis, a vaguely heritable and occult predisposition for chronic diseases such as TB. Having a diathesis required 'obey[ing] the whole physical and moral code', in the words of one American doctor.[55] By extension, the working classes, being at greater risk of illness and impairment owing to their nutritional state, living and working conditions and, as many middle-class individuals believed, poorly controlled behaviour, would have been perceived as having an even greater reason than the middle classes to maintain 'healthy' middle-class standards of behaviour. Indeed, patients were expected to have assessed their own risk of illness and responded accordingly. For example, of Francis M, introduced earlier, GRI medical staff disapprovingly commented that 'although he knew that his stomach was weak, he never restricted his diet'.[56]

By the latter half of the nineteenth century it was clear to concerned middle-class observers that neither medical science nor social reform had succeeded in improving the moral and physical health of the working classes, resulting in pessimism regarding the mission of charitable medical care. Fothergill lamented, 'If the artisan would but take somewhat more care of himself, his death rate would not be nearly so high, but how he is to be brought to see this, it is not so easy to say.'[57] Medical men more broadly criticised the largesse of the voluntary hospitals. An anonymous writer to *The Lancet* characterised the large number of patients treated in London charitable dispensaries and hospitals as 'ill-conceived prodigality which apes the name of Benevolence', stating categorically that 'It is not possible that one-tenth of the population are entitled to this gratuitous service.'[58] D. Campbell Black, a Glasgow surgeon, echoed Dickens' Ebenezer Scrooge in his exhortation to 'Stop this [hospital] charity and the working man will not be poor, he will not be improvident, and he will not be drunken ... and the parochial board, the only defensible form of charity, will be otherwise employed than in begetting pauperism, black-guardism, and crime.'[59]

Moral and physical degeneration in the British population were obsessions for the late-Victorians.[60] Critically, during this period, moral and physical degeneracy were linked as a single issue. British thinking on evolution was strongly flavoured by the Lamarckian inheritance of acquired characteristics, emphasising the contribution of behaviour.[61] Authors such as Fothergill described, for middle-class readers, a vicious cycle in which industrial labour drove workers to seek mental stimulation in 'drunkenness, political and theological agitation, bursts of excitement, and a sensational literature of the lowest order'.[62] This in turn meant that they required their children's labour in order to afford such pursuits.[63] Child labour, thus necessitated by immorality, led to physical degeneration. Fothergill believed that 'Sustained toil … at an early age … exercises a most deleterious influence over the processes of growth, as the stunted and ungainly figures of the manufacturing districts amply demonstrate.'[64] For Fothergill and others in the late-Victorian period, immorality and ill health were inextricably linked and imminently threatening to the nation's future.

Owing to the parallel drawn by the Scottish Enlightenment between the health of individuals and the health of the social body, the expectation that individuals should maintain or regain health would have been considered a responsibility not only to oneself but also to the nation.[65] This harks back to the contribution made by the productive working classes to national wealth, discussed above; and indeed the stigmatisation of working-class individuals with impairments becomes all too clear when one considers Enlightenment-era recommendations for the cure of the physical body alongside metaphors for the social body. William Cullen (1710–90), an RIE professor of medicine, is quoted by Stott as having written in an unpublished 1770 manuscript that 'our fluids are constantly Degenerating, and if they are not thrown out of the body they would soon be noxious to it'.[66]

The reformer the Reverend Andrew Mearns (1837–1925), in his 1883 'plain recital of plain facts' regarding the London poor, acknowledged that 'those who endeavour to earn their bread by honest work far outnumber the dishonest', but his nonetheless describing the subjects of his work as 'repulsive', 'depraved', 'dissolute' and 'drunken' revealed – in addition to an inordinate fondness for adjectives beginning with 'd' – his abhorrence at those whom he proposed to aid.[67] Mearns wrote of 'the misery inherited [by poor children] from the vice of drunken and dissolute parents … manifest in the stunted, misshapen, and often loathsome objects that we constantly meet'.[68] If physical degeneration, following Cullen, produced a noxious element that must be cast out to maintain the health of the body as a whole, what must be the parallel solution to social degeneration, of which illness and impairment among the working classes were regarded as symptoms? It is through such body–society metaphors that Engels' 'maimed' individuals appear 'loathsome' to Mearns and his contemporaries; that the failure to be 'cured' at voluntary hospitals like GRI and the RIE becomes not a medical failure but a personal failure to live within, or return to, middle-class norms of behaviour and health.[69]

'Fit person[s] for the enjoyment of the charity of the hospital'[70]

The interests of the Victorian middle classes included the well-being of the working classes and were marked by the former's emphasis on class distinctions. As the Victorian era progressed, membership in the middle classes came to rely less upon economic and professional standards and was increasingly defined by social and cultural traits, including moral restraint, personal responsibility and industriousness.[71] Public-mindedness also contributed to the zealous efforts of the middle classes to 'improve' the poor through endeavours that included charity hospitals and sanitary reform.[72] For middle-class reformers, improvement in the behaviour as well as the living conditions of the working classes was necessary. Social reformer Edwin Chadwick (1800–90), for example, emphasised the contribution of poor sanitary infrastructure to the high incidence of disease in working-class neighbourhoods. He also presented these neighbourhoods as sites of moral deterioration, describing instances in which working-class women did not maintain middle-class standards of cleanliness, despite having 'been taught the habits of neatness' or having 'received a very excellent ... moral education'.[73]

As a result of increasingly behaviour-driven definitions of the economically and socially powerful Victorian middle classes, behaviourally defined 'respectability' gained salience within charitable institutions like GRI and the RIE during the Victorian period. Conformity to hegemonically appropriate behaviour was expected, and its absence, real or presumed, was noted. At GRI this often took the form of commentary by medical staff regarding patients' 'deviant' behaviour and its implicit contribution to their disorders. By contrast, this style of comment is absent from GRI patient records for the pre-Victorian period (no patient records are preserved from the RIE prior to 1845).

Simply, behaviour outside of middle-class norms led medical staff to implicitly doubt patients' accounts on other points. Mary R, an 1855 phthisis patient at the RIE, 'states that she has always been well-fed and well-kept, and little exposed [to the elements]', all of which were indications of the careful self-maintenance of health espoused by the middle classes.[74] '[B]ut', the journal entry goes on to note, 'she is reputed as a femme du pavé', or prostitute, information evidently included in order to negate Mary R's own testimony.[75] The point at issue is not whether the patient was a prostitute; she may have engaged in sexual labour. Nor is it whether she was well-fed; to the contrary, medical staff noted that she was 'tolerably healthy looking and well-nourished'.[76] Rather, because she was said by an unnamed source to be a prostitute, her own account of healthy living was suspect, despite her healthy, well-nourished appearance.

The link between patients' behaviour and their health was also made explicit by senior medical colleagues, increasingly from the mid-Victorian period and later. The onset of RIE patient Andrew M's phthisis in 1855 was linked by medical staff to what they noted as a drunken 'debauch' and 'spree'.[77] Similarly, John R's phthisis originated in a cold caught in January 1859, 'while attending Burn's [sic, Robert Burns (1759–96)] centenary, having stood in cold and got wet'. The journal entry goes on to add, 'He had been drinking all night.'[78]

The deviant behaviour of others could also result in a patient's disease. In 1855 RIE phthisis patient Catherine S reported that she first coughed blood after an incident in which her husband – 'a man of drunken habits', wrote the medical staff – 'abused her, took the bed clothes away and sold them'.[79] While John T, admitted to GRI for phthisis in 1893, cited a draughty office as the source of his illness, medical staff instead placed blame with the patient's wife and housekeeper: 'Owing to the intemperance of his wife, has been separated from her ... He has been much neglected in consequence, careless housekeeper, badly cooked food, et cetera and this may have to do with his present condition.'[80]

Patients were expected to acknowledge the social distinction between themselves and those providing care through grateful submission to medical staff and hospital rules. Failure to do so was deeply disapproved, as in the case of Alexander D, an RIE phthisis patient in 1865. Alexander D 'was recommended ... as a fit person for the enjoyment of the charity of the hospital and was admitted because so recommended ... The patient, however, absconded before his case was properly taken'.[81] That the patient remained at the RIE for four days without having his case taken is not emphasised by the indignant staff member reporting Alexander D's unauthorised departure.

Through such cases, the medical staff at GRI and the RIE made clear their distaste for those violating behavioural expectations. In implicitly and explicitly connecting patients' ill health to their own and their relations' behaviour, medical staff linked working-class disease to deviance from middle-class norms. The middle-class medical staff did not make such connections between deviance and illness only in circumstances when their working-class patients did not, as in the cases of Andrew M and John R. Practitioners also made these connections when the patient attributed his illness to another cause, as for John T, and indeed when the practitioner's own observations confirmed the patient's account, as for Mary R. This middle-class prejudice established deviance as a cause of the increased prevalence of ill health and impairment among the working classes, and underscored the biological as well as social importance of respectability, while simultaneously placing blame with the working classes for their condition. At the same time, middle-class medical practitioners established themselves as, in addition to providers of healthcare, arbiters of healthy behaviour. By denying care to those deemed insufficiently respectable, the medical establishment further placed themselves as gatekeepers of restoration to health.

Conclusions

The living and working environments of working-class Victorians placed them at greater risk of illness and physical impairment than their contemporaries of higher socio-economic status. Owing to the class distinctions emphasised by the socially and economically powerful middle classes, however, treatment of such conditions among the working classes commonly relied on charitable medical establishments, access to which was regulated. For GRI and the RIE, the 'worthy poor' to whom admission was extended were expected to conform to middle-class behavioural norms, including productive labour. Attempts to restrict the admission of those with incurable disorders, who thus were not expected to return to work, revealed a connection between health status and social status. Specifically, the ability to engage in productive labour contributed socially as well as economically to social status. It was this interplay between marginalised statuses – illness/impairment and membership of the working classes – that fed the stigmatisation of impairment in its modern form.

The importance of work in defining ability and respectability, together with the self-defined role of the middle classes – and middle-class medical practitioners in particular – as arbiters and gatekeepers of health, acted to exclude individuals with impairments from both respectability and the voluntary hospital healthcare that might allow their 'reclamation' under Victorian hegemony. This circular mechanism of exclusion engendered social disability through the lens of medical disability. The disillusionment of early and mid-Victorian reformers with their failed efforts to restore individuals with impairments was harnessed in the late-Victorian period into the reclassification of many working-class invalids as refractory, unfit for the charity of voluntary hospitals and incapable of restoration to industry and usefulness, thereby constructing impairment as discrediting for generations to come.

Notes

1 See, for example, P. Joshi, 'Edwin Chadwick's self-fashioning: professionalism, masculinity, and the Victorian poor', *Victorian Literature and Culture*, 32:2 (2004), 353–70.

2 See, for example, the work of Edwin Chadwick, Hector Gavin, Thomas Southwood Smith and the Health of Towns Association: E. Chadwick, *Report on the Sanitary Condition of the Labouring Population of Great Britain: A Supplementary Report on*

the Results of a Special Inquiry Into the Practice of Interment in Towns [1843] (reprint) (Edinburgh: Edinburgh University Press, 1965); H. Gavin, *Unhealthiness of London, and the Necessity of Remedial Measures* [1847] and *The Habitations of the Industrial Classes: Their Influence on the Physical and on the Social and Moral Condition of these Classes* [1850] (reprints) in L. H. Lees and A. Lees (eds), *The Rise of Urban Britain: A Collection of Thirty-Five Important Titles Documenting this Major Transformation and the Responses to It* (New York, NY: Garland Publishing Inc, 1985); R. G. Paterson, 'The Health of Towns Association in Great Britain 1844–1849', *Bulletin of the History of Medicine*, 22 (1948), 373–402; T. S. Smith, *Results of Sanitary Improvement, Illustrated by the Operation of the Metropolitan Societies for Improving the Dwellings of the Industrious Classes, the Working of the Common Lodging-Houses Act, Etc.* (London: Charles Knight, 1854).

3   F. Engels, *The Condition of the Working-Class in England*, trans. Florence Kelley Wischnewetzky [1844] (reprint) (London: Swan Sonnenschein & Co, 1892); R. Dubos and J. Dubos, *The White Plague: Tuberculosis, Man, and Society* [1952] (reprint) (New Brunswick, NJ: Rutgers University Press, 1996); B. Haley, *The Healthy Body and Victorian Culture* (Cambridge, MA: Harvard University Press, 1978).

4   For discussion of adoption of the stethoscope at GRI, see A. W. Farnbach Pearson, 'Tuberculosis, Social Inequality, and the Hospital in Nineteenth-century Scotland' (PhD thesis, Arizona State University, 2013), chapter 4; for Edinburgh, see M. Nicolson, 'The introduction of percussion and stethoscopy to early nineteenth-century Edinburgh', in W. F. Bynum and R. Porter (eds), *Medicine and the Five Senses* (Cambridge: Cambridge University Press, 1993), pp. 134–53.

5   For example, R. T. H. Laënnec, *De L'Auscultation Médiate; ou Traité du Diagnostic des Maladies des Poumons et du Coeur, Fondé Principalement Sur ce Nouveau Moyen D'Exploration* (Paris: J-A. Brosson et J-S. Chaudé, 1819).

6   D. Porter and R. Porter, *Patient's Progress: Doctors and Doctoring in Eighteenth-century England* (Stanford, CA: Stanford University Press, 1989).

7   See, for example, M. A. Crowther and M. W. Dupree, *Medical Lives in the Age of Surgical Revolution* (Cambridge: Cambridge University Press, 2007).

8   J. A. Jenkinson, 'A "crutch to assist in gaining an honest living": dispensary shopkeeping by Scottish general practitioners and the responses of the British medical elite, ca. 1852–1911', *Bulletin of the History of Medicine*, 86:1 (2012), 1–36.

9   Greater Glasgow and Clyde Health Board Archive (hereafter GGCHBA), HB14/2/4, GRI Annual Report 1835, p. 5.

10   T. N. Bonner, *Becoming a Physician: Medical Education in Great Britain, France, Germany, and the United States 1750–1945* (Oxford: Oxford University Press, 1995), p. 43.

11   A. L. Turner, *Story of a Great Hospital: The Royal Infirmary of Edinburgh 1729–1929* [1937] (reprint) (Edinburgh: The Mercat Press, 1979).

12   Jenkinson, 'Crutch', 6.

13   *Ibid.*, 16.

14   R. Richardson, *Death, Dissection and the Destitute*, 2nd edn (London: Phoenix Press, 1988), p. 275.

15 For GRI, see GGCHBA, HH67/56 series, Admission and Discharge Registers, 1837–1901; for RIE, see Lothian Health Services Archive (hereafter LHSA), LHB1/126 series, Admission and Discharge Registers, 1837–1901.

16 See, for example, Dubos and Dubos, *White Plague*; D. S. Barnes, *The Making of a Social Disease: Tuberculosis in Nineteenth-Century France* (Berkeley, CA: University of California Press, 1995).

17 Engels, *Condition of the Working-Class*, p. 164.

18 For discussion of the development and implications of this legislation, see Richardson, *Death, Dissection and the Destitute*.

19 See, for example, J. H. Bennett, *The Pathology and Treatment of Pulmonary Tuberculosis; and on the Local Medication of Pharyngeal and Laryngeal Diseases Frequently Mistaken for, or Associated With, Phthisis* (Edinburgh: Sutherland and Knox, 1853), p. 51.

20 M. Brown, '"Like a devoted army": Medicine, heroic masculinity, and the military paradigm in Victorian Britain', *Journal of British Studies*, 49:3 (2010), 592–622; Chadwick, *Supplementary Report*; Gavin, *Unhealthiness of London*; Joshi, 'Edwin Chadwick'; Haley, *Healthy Body*, p. 6.

21 Chadwick, *Supplementary Report*; Gavin, *Habitations of the Industrial Classes*; J. E. Paluzzi, 'A social disease/a social response: Lessons in tuberculosis from early 20th century Chile', *Social Science & Medicine*, 59 (2004), pp. 763–73; T. H. C. Stevenson, 'The vital statistics of wealth and poverty', *Journal of the Royal Statistical Society*, 91: 2 (1928), 207–30.

22 J. H. Bennett, *Treatise on the Oleum Jecoris Aselli, or Cod Liver Oil, as a Therapeutic Agent in Certain Forms of Gout, Rheumatism, and Scrofula: With Cases* (London: S. Highley, 1841).

23 Bennett, *Pathology and Treatment*, p. 52.

24 F. W. Burton-Fanning, *The Open-Air Treatment of Pulmonary Tuberculosis*, 2nd ed. (London: Cassell & Co, 1909); see also A. Latham, 'Essay on the erection of a sanatorium for the treatment of tuberculosis in England', *Lancet*, 1:4140 (1903), 3–42; A. Latham, *The Diagnosis and Modern Treatment of Pulmonary Consumption* (New York, NY: William Wood & Co, 1907), p. 81; J. H. Pratt, 'The "home sanatorium" treatment of consumption', *Boston Medical and Surgical Journal*, 154:8 (1906), 210–16.

25 Engels, *Condition of the Working-Class*, p. 164.

26 *Ibid.*

27 LHSA, LHB1/1/13, RIE Minutes of Managers' Meetings, 1844, p. 507.

28 C. Gallagher, 'The body versus the social body in the works of Thomas Malthus and Henry Mayhew', *Representations* 14 (1986), 83–106.

29 T. Percival, *Medical Ethics: Or, a Code of Institutes and Precepts, Adapted to the Professional Conduct of Physicians and Surgeons* (Manchester: S. Russell for J. Johnson, 1803), pp. 17–18.

30 *Ibid.*

31 *Ibid.*

32 *Ibid.*, p. 127.

33   GGCHBA, HB14/5/13, GRI Journal of Female Ward, April to November 1798, front matter, p. 54.

34   LHSA, LHB1/129/5/44, RIE Journal of Ward 11, 1865, p. 62.

35   LHSA, LHB1/1/19, RIE Minutes of the Managers' Meetings 1855, p. 7.

36   For example, LHSA, LHB1/1/13, RIE Minutes of the Managers' Meetings 1844, p. 500; GGCHBA, HB14/1/14, GRI Minutes of the Managers' Meetings 1875, p. 175.

37   LHSA, LHB1/1/13, RIE Minutes of the Managers' Meetings 1844, p. 506.

38   GGCHBA, HB14/1/3, GRI Annual Report 1815, p. 153.

39   LHSA, LHB1/1/13, RIE Minutes of the Managers' Meetings 1844, p. 507.

40   *Ibid.*, p. 508.

41   *Ibid.*

42   *Ibid.*, pp. 506–9.

43   *Ibid.*, p. 509.

44   Richardson, *Death, Dissection and the Destitute.*

45   J. H. Bennett, *Clinical Lectures on the Principles and Practice of Medicine* (New York, NY: Samuel S. & William Wood, 1858), p. 25.

46   LHSA, LHB1/4/80, RIE Annual Report 1880/81, p. 19.

47   LHSA, LHB1/4/84, RIE Annual Report 1884/85, p. 17.

48   GGCHBA, HH67/12/20, GRI Ward Journal 1905, p. 353.

49   R. Noyes Jr, 'The transformation of hypochondriasis in British medicine, 1680–1830', *Social History of Medicine*, 24:2 (2011), 293.

50   T. Parsons, *The Social System* (Glencoe, IL: The Free Press, 1951).

51   Mearns, *Bitter Cry.*

52   Compare with S. L. Gilman, *Difference and Pathology: Stereotypes of Sexuality, Race, and Madness* (Ithaca, NY: Cornell University Press, 1985).

53   J. Rosenberg, 'The bitter fruit: heredity, disease, and social thought in nineteenth-century America', *Perspectives in American History* 8 (1974), 189–235.

54   J. M. Fothergill, *The Maintenance of Health: A Medical Work for Lay Readers* (London: Smith, Elder & Co, 1874), pp. 24–5.

55   W. A. Alcott, *The Laws of Health* (Boston, MA: John P Jewett and Company, 1857), p. 13.

56   GGCHBA, HH67/12/20, GRI Ward Journal, 1905, p. 353.

57   Fothergill, *Maintenance of Health*, p. 69.

58   Anonymous, 'Where to draw the line', *Lancet*, 70:1788 (1857), 586.

59   D. C. Black, 'Special hospitals', *Lancet*, 100:2550 (1872), 60.

60   For example, B. Luckin, 'Revisiting the idea of degeneration in urban Britain, 1830–1900', *Urban History*, 33:2 (2006), 234–52; Rosenberg, 'The bitter fruit'; P. Pinell, 'Degeneration theory and heredity patterns between 1850 and 1900', in J-P. Gaudillière and I. Löwy (eds), *Heredity and Infection: The History of Disease Transmission* (London: Routledge, 2001), pp. 245–59; G. S. Jones, *Outcast London: A Study in the Relationship between Classes in Victorian Society* (Oxford: Clarendon Press, 1971).

61 P. J. Bowler, *Evolution: The History of an Idea*, 25th anniversary edition (Berkeley, CA: University of California Press, 2009), pp. 236–40.

62 Fothergill, *Maintenance of Health*, p. 65.

63 *Ibid.*, p. 48.

64 *Ibid.*

65 Gallagher, 'The body versus the social body'.

66 Quoted in R. Stott, 'Health and virtue: Or, how to keep out of harm's way. Lectures on pathology and therapeutics by William Cullen c. 1770', *Medical History*, 31:2 (1987), 132.

67 A. Mearns, *The Bitter Cry of Outcast London: An Inquiry Into the Condition of the Abject Poor* (London: James Clarke & Co, 1883).

68 *Ibid.*

69 Engels, *Condition of the Working-Class*, p. 164.

70 LHSA, LHB1/129/2/57, RIE Journal of Ward, 1 June 1864 to July 1865, p. 206.

71 S. Gunn, 'Class, identity and the urban: the middle class in England, c. 1790–1950', *Urban History*, 31:1 (2004), 36; also see J. E. Butler, *Social Purity*, 1879 (Reprint) (Victorian Women Writers Project, http://purl.dlib.indiana.edu/iudl/vwwp/VAB7160, 2007); Mearns, *Bitter Cry*.

72 Brown, 'Like a devoted army'; Joshi, 'Edwin Chadwick'.

73 E. Chadwick, *Report to Her Majesty's Principal Secretary of State for the Home Department, From the Poor Law Commissioners, on an Inquiry into the Sanitary Condition of the Labouring Population of Great Britain* (London: W Clowes and Sons, 1842), pp. 127–9.

74 Alcott, *Laws of Health*, p. 13; Fothergill, *Maintenance of Health*, pp. 24–5; LHSA, LHB1/129/5/22, RIE Journal of Ward, 11 August 1855 to February 1856, p. 105; Rosenberg, 'The bitter fruit'.

75 LHSA, LHB1/129/5/22, RIE Journal of Ward, 11 August 1855 to February 1856, p. 105.

76 *Ibid.*, p. 106.

77 LHSA, LHB1/129/2/54, RIE Journal of Ward, 1 June 1855 to September 1855, p. 167.

78 LHSA, LHB1/129/2/26, RIE Journal of Ward, 1 November 1859 to October 1860, p. 91.

79 LHSA, LHB1/129/5/22, RIE Journal of Ward, 11 August 1855 to February 1856, p. 55.

80 GGCHBA, HH67/7/5, GRI Ward Journal, 1893, p. 200.

81 LHSA, LHB1/129/2/57, RIE Journal of Ward, 1 June 1864 to July 1865, p. 206.

2

IMPERIAL LIVES: CONFRONTING THE LEGACIES OF EMPIRE, DISABILITY AND THE VICTORIANS

Esme Cleall

This chapter explores the life histories of three deaf men and women from nineteenth-century Britain: John Kitto (1804–54), George Tait (1828–1904) and Jane Groom (1839–1918), who all can, in some ways, be said to have lived imperial lives. John Kitto, from Plymouth, started work as a missionary in Malta and later travelled to Baghdad where he wrote several texts in the 'Orientalist' vein. George Tait, born in the Scottish Highlands, became a Canadian settler and set up the first school for the deaf in Halifax, Nova Scotia. Jane Groom, originally from Shropshire, tried to establish a 'deaf colony' in Canada using the 1872 Homestead Act, which directly dispossessed First Nations people to secure land. As the lives of these three individuals intersected with the workings of the British Empire, this gives us an opportunity to consider the intersection between disability and colonialism more broadly.

Scholars of disability have often used the language of colonialism to evoke the exclusion, discrimination and subjugation of disabled people by society. In 1977 T. Szasz used the expression 'psychiatric slavery' to sum up the containment of mental health patients in American institutions: a stark image suggestive of violence, forced labour and alienation as well as 'unfreedom'.[1] More recently, Karen Hirsch, writing of the historical treatment of disabled people in the United States, has used the language of colonialism to describe a past where disabled people were treated as second-class citizens.[2] Meanwhile, Goggin and Newell have discussed the situation of disabled people in contemporary Australia as being one of 'apartheid', not least due to the elements of social segregation, political isolation and economic marginalisation at stake.[3] A similar tactic has been to deploy the language of race – intimately bound up, as race is, with processes of colonialism and imperialism – to suggest the way in which disabled people have been, and continue to be, stigmatised. Leonard Kreigal most famously made this case when he discussed 'the cripple as Negro' in British and American fiction.[4] While these arguments have been made of a range of physical and mental disabilities, the construction of disabled people as 'colonised' has perhaps been made most strongly by Deaf activists and scholars. Harlan Lane, among others, has used the parity between the suppression of sign language and the suppression of indigenous spoken languages to claim members of Deaf cultures as a linguistic and cultural minority suffering the 'physical subjugation of a disempowered people, the imposition of alien language and mores, and the regulation of education on behalf of the colonizer's goals'.[5]

The use of colonial, postcolonial and racial imagery by disabled activists and scholars has been important in helping us to understand the dire treatment of disabled people and the multiple layers at which the subordination of disabled people has occurred. It is not simply that disabled people have been stigmatised or unable to work because of the social response to impairment; rather, an ableist agenda has constructed them as utterly 'other', where discrimination has become systematic.[6] This has made the tools provided by postcolonial studies scholars to explore the concept of alterity highly important in helping to examine the construction of disability. As I have argued elsewhere, the construction of the colonial 'other' and the demarcation of those deemed to be 'disabled' were not only parallel developments but related ones.[7] In the nineteenth century, as both the languages of 'race' and the languages of 'disability' hardened, the construction of each category of difference became interrelated: they were part and parcel of the same discursive process.

However, an overly simplistic use of postcolonial imagery to convey, explain and evoke disability does have significant limitations. For one thing, it is potentially reductive and distortive. Disabled people and people deemed not to be 'white' may both have been subordinated by the major European empires, at home and overseas, but the methods in which each was marginalised from an able, white society were very different and had very different consequences for each. Furthermore, as Mark Sherry has argued, there is the danger that analytically conflating these two categories of difference not only confuses but actually obscures the history of both disabled people and people who were colonised.[8] One history that it marginalises in particular is that of disabled people who might have identified themselves, or been identified by others, as colonisers. In nineteenth-century Britain, when the British Empire was a huge part of British society, culture, politics and economics, it may well have been that imperialism shaped the lives of disabled people both as colonisers and, we might argue, as colonised.

In this chapter I ask whether disabled people themselves participated in colonial practices. It would be surprising if they did not. In the nineteenth century perceived racial difference was used to justify the transatlantic slave trade, the expropriation of indigenous land across Australasia, Africa and the Americas, and violence of genocidal proportion in Tasmania. The colonial 'other' became a subject of ethnographic examination, pseudo-scientific investigation, literary curiosity, political subjugation, economic exploitation, Christianising mission and philanthropic crusade. Imperialism infiltrated British culture in complex and manifold ways, from high politics, to education, to literature. Suffusing British culture as it did, imperialism brought with it increased sensitivity to questions of race, nationhood and belonging – at home as well as overseas.[9] While different social groups had different levels of involvement in the British Empire, an argument has been made that imperialism affected all men and women back in metropolitan Britain, whether that was in forging the iron shackles that bound the enslaved, weaving cotton exported by the East India Company, or consuming the sugar grown on West Indian plantations.

The aim of this chapter is certainly not to condemn Kitto, Tait and Groom by naming them as 'imperialists' and consigning them to a 'dirty' past. Nor is the aim to claim that they, in many ways extraordinary individuals, were representative of all deaf and/or disabled people. The point is simply to think about what happens to our ideas and understandings of disability when we use an imperial rather than a national framework; to think about what happens when disabled people also occupy positions of relative power; and what happened when there was a slippage, which many today would find uneasy, between disability and colonialism. Tait, Kitto and Groom differ as individuals and in their experiences of empire and of deafness, but I believe that looking at them together helps us to think about the diversity of colonial experiences, as well as reclaiming the lives of deaf people, who, when not marginalised altogether, are most often confined within the history of victimhood.

John Kitto (1804–54)

The first of my case studies is John Kitto, a deaf man from a working-class family in Plymouth.[10] Born hearing, Kitto became deaf at the age of twelve when he fell thirty-five feet from a roof on to the paved courtyard below, sustaining considerable injury to his head. Regaining consciousness after a two-week coma, Kitto found that not only had he lost his hearing, but his voice had become painful and hard to use, while his enunciation, which had previously been 'remarkably clear and distinct', had become 'much altered' and difficult to understand.[11] His deafness thus manifested in the visible marker of having to use the manual alphabet to spell out what he wanted to say, though he distanced himself from the wider deaf community, claiming to have always 'abominated' sign language, which he considered beneath him.[12] Social class as well as disability shaped Kitto's early experiences. He came from a family deeply impoverished due to his father's alcoholism, and he spent his childhood and adolescence in and out of workhouses.

Kitto's first engagement with the British Empire came from his role as a missionary for the evangelical Church Missionary Society (CMS), under whose auspices he travelled to Malta in June 1827. At that time, Malta occupied the unusual position of being a British colony in the Mediterranean. The relationship between missionaries and imperialism is very complicated and varied greatly over time and place.[13] Some historians have suggested that the 'Bible followed the flag', shoring up a British presence in distant colonial spaces, while others have drawn attention to points at which the relationship between missionaries and the colonial state was actively antagonistic.[14] But, whatever the correlation with the formal British Empire, it is clear that missionaries were agents of cultural imperialism. It was not simply that missionaries encouraged the proselytisation of indigenous people in and beyond the Empire, but that they engaged in a widespread process of cultural reform, demanding that prospective converts should adopt a wide range of Western behaviours. These included embracing 'civilisation' through certain forms of dress, living quarters that focused on providing personal privacy and the curtailment of polygamous marriages.[15] For this reason Jeffrey Cox, among others, has raised the question as to whether Protestant missionaries were in fact the 'worst imperialists of them all', more penetrative into indigenous cultures than 'official' colonial activity.[16]

While race and gender have now been widely recognised as structuring the missionary world, so too were they ableist enterprises that privileged the non-disabled body.[17] One way in which this can be seen is through their use of language and imagery. Missionaries consistently characterised non-Christian peoples ('heathens' in the contemporary language) through the imagery of disability, claiming that Indians and Africans, among other colonial people, were 'deaf to the word', 'blind to the light' and 'too lame to walk alone'.[18]

A second way in which the missionary enterprise was structured by ableism can be seen in its recruitment policies. Highly conscious of the costs of supporting incapacitated missionaries, and saturated with their own prejudices around mental, physical and spiritual 'health', missionary societies throughout this period systematically filtered out those deemed to have a physical or emotional impairment. In the London Missionary Society, candidates who had experienced, or had a family history of, epilepsy or mental illness were automatically rejected, as were those who had speech impediments, who were deaf or who had a family history of deafness – conditions believed to impede a candidate's ability to learn a foreign language.[19] It was perhaps for these reasons that, when it was first suggested, Kitto saw a missionary career as an impossibility: 'I thought myself entirely incompetent to the duties of so arduous a station', and he considered his 'deafness' an 'obstacle'. However in this case a solution was found whereby he worked for the Church Missionary Society (a major, Anglican missionary organisation) as a printer.[20]

Ableism can also be seen in the way in which Kitto was treated by the CMS when he was in Malta. Kitto had a series of disagreements with the other missionaries in Malta, not least because, due to his deafness, he found it difficult to join in their evening conversations and preferred to spend the time reading alone, something that was not considered acceptable in this particular missionary circle where part of being a 'good colleague' involved shared socialising. He left Malta on bad terms with his employers, complaining that they did not understand his 'privations' as a deaf man who found communication difficult.

As a printer, rather than as an evangelist, Kitto was one step removed from the people of Malta, but nonetheless he was deeply implicated in the cultural imperialism of the missionary enterprise, printing the texts used for converting people to Protestantism and supporting the infrastructure of the CMS enterprise in Malta. Furthermore, his writing about Malta demonstrates that, along with his hearing colleagues, Kitto was imbued in the prejudices of wider missionary discourse and was shocked and disturbed by the Catholicism he encountered. 'The people of this island are very zealous,' he wrote in a private letter to friends back home, 'but it is the zeal of error against truth, of darkness against light.'[21]

It is for his second colonial encounter, in the Middle East, where he travelled as the tutor of the children of missionary Anthony Groves (1795–1853), that Kitto is more widely known, as his journal, 'The Deaf Traveller', was published upon his return in *The Penny Magazine*. Kitto visited Baghdad during a period of extreme political turbulence and his arrival in 1830 shortly preceded three major occurrences: the dispossession of the Mamluk rulers and reimposition of direct Ottoman rule by Ali Ridha Pasha (1864–1943), a protracted siege and an outbreak of plague. While, unlike Malta, Baghdad was not a site of formal British control in this period, there were ways in which a colonising European influence was starting to be felt, including through the presence of an East India Company Resident in the city and the missionary work of Kitto's employer and others.[22]

In Baghdad, Kitto clearly identified himself in the position of the white coloniser, and unlike the 'natives' he encountered in the street and in the marketplace. Interestingly, as I have explored elsewhere, in this location Kitto's Europeanness also worked to counteract some of the manifestations of his deafness.[23] In Baghdad, neither his laboured articulation nor his occasional resort to gesture, of which Kitto was usually very self-conscious, was an identifiable performance of deafness. While bemoaning his powers of articulation in Britain, which he claimed induced people to stop and stare at him, in Baghdad Kitto believed that his occasional signing caused him 'to seem to them rather as a foreigner ignorant of their language, than as deaf; and the resort to signs had not strangeness to them or attracted that notice from others which it never fails to do in this country [Britain]'.[24]

Even more identifiable performances of deafness, such as finger-spelling, could be represented in the colonial field not as disability, but as one of the wondrous European 'achievements' brought to un-European spaces. Of finger-spelling or the manual alphabet Kitto wrote:

> How greatly did not ... the natives of the country marvel at it, as one of the mysteries which might have been hidden under the seal of Solomon. And how pleasant was it to behold the reverence and admiration of THE USEFUL eradiate their swart countenances when the simple principle of the art was explained to them, and it was shown to be as available FOR THEIR OWN LANGUAGES – Arabian, Persian, Turkish – as for any other.[25]

Here, finger-spelling is imbued with the same awe-inspiring powers that missionaries described the written word to have had in other contexts. Finger-spelling was not represented here as a signifier of disability, but as another example of the enlightened technology of the European.[26]

As Edward Said and other postcolonial writers have identified, one of the key ways in which Europeans constructed 'the West' as superior to 'the East' was through writing about the East in an 'orientalising' manner: constructing it as mystical, exotic, but ultimately 'different'. Kitto's reading of Baghdad as 'the great scene of Arabian Tale and romance' can be placed in this tradition.[27] So too can his later works, written when he had returned to England, and which included: *The Pictorial Bible*, published in three large volumes between 1835 and 1838; *History of Palestine and the Holy Land, including a Complete History of the Jews* (two volumes, 1841); *History of Palestine from the Patriarchal Age to the Present Time* (1852); *Cyclopaedia of Biblical Literature* (two volumes, 1848).

Kitto's narratives are full of the details one might expect from any piece of travel writing from the Middle East: trials with packhorses, the 'strange' people, landscapes and customs he encounters, the intrigue with which the 'Arabs and the Turks' treated his lead pencil; and exciting illustrations of camels and turbaned men.[28] Kitto writes from an essentially European perspective, making many observations, on behalf of his imagined European readers, about the perceived bodily 'difference' of the Oriental 'natives', and how they could sit cross-legged for long periods without pain and bear high degrees of thirst.[29] As in the accounts of contemporary 'Orientalist' writers, Kitto's whiteness, masculinity, learning and familiarity through travel with the places about which he is writing, combine to create the authoritative voice typical of a colonial writer. Characteristic tropes include his 'ethnographic' descriptions of place and people, and the collapsing of space and time in depictions of the 'East' where the assumption is made that by looking at Palestine and Persia in the 1830s one would 'see' the 'Biblical Land' of two millennia earlier.[30]

Through writing about the 'Orient', Kitto made quite a name for himself as a travel writer and biblical scholar. As such, he was able to distance himself from his deaf identity, which was carefully separated from his authorial identity. He was also able, to some degree, to escape his working-class roots and, while often short of money, was able to adopt a much more middle-class persona and lifestyle until his relatively early death at the age of fifty while travelling to Germany in search of a cure for the headaches that had plagued him since his initial accident.

George Tait (1828–1904)

George Tait had a quite different life trajectory to that of John Kitto, not least in terms of his relationship with the British Empire.[31] Tait was born in 1828 in Watten, a rural parish in the county of Caithness in the far north of Scotland. While rapidly becoming incorporated in the imperial metropole, the Highlands where Tait was born were still perceived by the dominant English culture as 'wild', 'clannish', 'uncivilised' and 'different'. Emerging from a prolonged programme of clearance of people from the land, the Highlands had witnessed a process of radical 'internal colonisation' in favour of sheep farming that propelled hundreds of thousands of Scots into the Empire as refugees, emigrants and settlers.[32]

Tait depicted his childhood, while rural and poor, in a way that seems idyllic compared to Kitto's experiences of poverty and deprivation: surrounded by loving parents, grandparents and younger siblings. It can be speculated – from the complete absence of further information – that Tait was born deaf; he certainly never mentions the cause of his condition. He writes of his deafness as a special gift: 'I had … a sort of vague idea that I was the only deaf and dumb person in the world, and I sigh as I remember those days of blissful ignorance when I knew nothing of this hard, cruel world.'[33] His parents, however, worried about his deafness and, when they moved to the town of Wick, were relieved to find out about deaf institutions. Tait was sent to a deaf institution in Edinburgh, a considerable distance from his home.

Tait was educated at the Edinburgh Institution for the Deaf and Dumb, a large and prestigious organisation that itself had imperial connections.[34] Fellow students came from various places across the Empire, including the Australian colonies, Cape Colony, Hudson's Bay, India, Ireland, Jamaica and the Orange Free State, and from the United States.[35] Students learned about places of empire through written exercises, and there was a considerable exchange of staff between Britain, the United States and Canada.[36] In his memoir Tait described a lively time at school filled with 'wild sports', 'pranks' and mischief with the other boys.[37] There seems to have been a great sense of comradery among the students, and perhaps a sense of affiliation born from the shared experience of deafness.

Like Kitto, Tait also had ambitions to travel. At the age of sixteen, and against the advice of his father, he left school early with his mind 'full of what I had heard about countries far across the sea' and with the intention of seeing the world.[38] After a brief stay in London, he travelled to France, then back to Liverpool where he was determined to fulfil his dream and travel to America, a place he saw as 'a bright vision of silver and gold' where he could 'make [his] fortune'.[39] When he eventually arrived in North America, Tait did not find his fortune, but worked on a shipyard on the East Coast. Learning of an uncle who had settled in Nova Scotia, Tait changed his plans and, following a brief correspondence, went to join him in Halifax; Tait eventually married and lived there for the remainder of his life.

Shortly after his arrival in Halifax, Tait was approached by the father of a twelve-year-old deaf girl who, until then, had received no education on account of her deafness. The father asked Tait to teach her. Education formed another link tying metropole and colony together, and it did so for the deaf as well as for the hearing. For example, settlers in New Zealand, Australia and Canada often sent their deaf children back to Britain for education where the institutions were more developed.[40] And teachers took with them new resources, information and pedagogical techniques. In Halifax, the girl's schooling soon attracted other deaf children from the vicinity and Tait began larger classes. Walking along the street one day, he noticed a man and woman conversing in sign-language. On approaching them, he discovered that the man, William Grey, had, like Tait himself, been educated at the Edinburgh Institution. They subsequently set up an institution in Halifax that grew in size, and they recruited additional teachers from Scotland.

Tait's only publication, his *Autobiography of a Deaf Mute*, was firmly located within a disabled identity. Not only is the book prefixed and suffixed by engravings of the 'deaf and dumb alphabet', but it is published alongside a general account of deaf education, tying together these issues. The main text of the book offers a short but lively narrative of Tait's life and the establishment of the Halifax

Institution. Another striking element of the text is that it is clear that Tait was writing from a colonial space and addressing a Canadian audience rather than a British one. His opening passage reads: 'To begin my history where my life began, I shall invite my reader to travel in imagination far across the broad Atlantic, to the heathery hill of "Auld Scotland" where the kilted lads are born.' The primary place through which the adult Tait constitutes his identity, therefore, is Halifax. Tait had become a settler.

Assessing Tait's engagement with concepts of empire is perhaps harder than it is in Kitto's case. Although, unlike Kitto, Tait did not write about the active performance of a 'white' identity, he nonetheless crossed spaces of empire and engaged, albeit often indirectly, in acts of colonial settlement. Canada was a place that saw the massive dispossession of indigenous people. And colonial settlement was a violent form of colonial conquest. As the theorist of colonial settlement Lorenzo Veracini argues, 'not all migrants are settlers', but settlers carry with them a distinct sovereign capacity; Tait became part of this ruling class, or ruling race.[41]

Jane Groom (1839–1918)[42]

Jane Groom was born of a higher social standing than either Tait or Kitto. Groom was firmly middle class, her father being a land surveyor and her mother a figure of some local influence. However, after her education in the Deaf and Dumb School in Old Trafford, Manchester, she moved to London and became deeply involved with the impoverished deaf community in the capital's East End. In some ways, Groom might be identified, using the colonial imagery I discussed at the beginning of this chapter, as a deaf 'compatrador', someone whom Deaf theorist Paddy Ladd describes as one of a 'small group of Deaf people, mostly of middle-class parentage', who allowed benevolently minded yet essentially disempowering hearing philanthropists to access the deaf in order to engage with a form of 'missionary colonialism'.[43] Certainly, Groom became tightly networked within a small group of hearing philanthropists and teachers concerned with deaf education and missionary work in East London, and particularly with the Reverend Samuel Smith (c. 1832–83) of the Association to Aid the Deaf and Dumb (AADD) and with the Reverend William Stainer (1828–98), his assistant. She worked for a while with females at the British Asylum for Deaf and Dumb and later became a 'teacher of deaf and dumb children' under the London School Board.[44]

Horrified by the poverty and destitution which she encountered in and around Bethnal Green, Groom looked for ways to improve the lives of people in London. After losing her job as a deaf teacher in the wake of the 1880 Milan

Conference, which, among other things, made it increasingly difficult for teachers who were themselves deaf to get employment teaching deaf children, she travelled to Canada in 1881.[45] In Manitoba she met two men whom she later claimed to have 'sent' there from the workhouse eighteen months previously. Both appeared to be doing 'exceedingly well', and much better than in London where unemployment was high and poverty was rife.[46]

From examining the cases of these two men, Groom proposed that a more formal arrangement should be established whereby deaf people from the East End could be moved to Manitoba, a Canadian province which was in the throes of colonisation. 'I have noticed so much distress among the deaf and dumb', she wrote, 'that I feel perfectly sad at witnessing it, and I am sure that nothing can be done for them here [in London] to establish them satisfactorily. My opinion on this subject is that the only scheme to accomplish their ultimate well-being is to carry out my scheme of emigration to Canada.'[47] What had started as the ad hoc relocation of a couple of deaf settlers and their families therefore became something larger. It became, as Groom herself put it, 'An Emigration Scheme for the Deaf and Dumb'. She set up the Deaf and Dumb Emigration Society, asking for contributions to be passed on to Richenda Fry (1808–84), a great-neice of Elizabeth Fry (1780–1845), and herself deaf. In 1884 Groom travelled to Canada again, this time with ten deaf men, intending to settle a 'colony' for the deaf in the Canadian North-West. Over the next ten years, Groom settled twenty-four more deaf settlers and their families in Canada, much to the outrage of local white settlers who claimed that the 'deaf mutes' would be unable to support themselves and would soon be reliant on charity.[48]

This was a period when there was much propaganda encouraging people to move to Canada, and which promoted Canada as having an abundance of resources and space. The indigenous peoples who owned and lived on the land were deliberately excluded from these representations. The Dominion Lands Act, or the 'Homestead' Act, which was passed in Canada in 1872, had stipulated that individual white settlers might be 'given' 164 hectares of indigenous land in what became Manitoba and the North-West Territories, partly in a bid to stop the land being colonised by the United States. First Nations people were never compensated for this land. Under the terms of the Dominion Lands Act, Jane Groom proposed that 'each deaf and dumb person with family shall receive from fifty to one hundred and sixty acres for cultivation and, if deserving, one hundred and sixty more, as provided in the offer to emigrants by the Canadian Government'.[49] In Britain, talks, pamphlets and meetings were used to attract settlers.

While the kinds of settlers that Canada wanted were essentially those who were white, able-bodied and British, various groups were able to use the legislation to their own ends, and this period saw the settlement of Mennonite and Jewish communities in Manitoba as well as schemes for utopias, such as that envisaged by the Church Colonisation Society. Sir Charles Tupper (1821–1915), who later became Canada's shortest-serving prime minister, was High Commissioner of Canada in London from 1883 to 1895 and was active in encouraging emigration to Canada.[50] Among other things, he engaged in considerable correspondence about Jane Groom and her scheme, forwarding a copy of her pamphlet, *A Future for the Deaf and Dumb in the Canadian North West*, to the Department of Agriculture in Canada.[51]

In order to engage with Groom's life and experiences, we must recognise that hers was a life profoundly shaped by imperial dynamics. Groom experienced many hardships on account of her deafness, her loss of employment following the Conference of Milan being a particularly stark example. But she was also able to benefit from her status as a white, middle-class woman in imperial Britain. Groom exuded confidence in her dealings with colonial officials when writing to the Department of Agriculture, the government department most associated with the Homesteader scheme, and she secured funding from, among others, William Gladstone via the secretive Royal Bounty Fund.[52]

The Canadian Government held an ambivalent position in relation to the settlers. While several historians have usefully elucidated the way in which colonial governments were often very hostile to disabled settlers, and while the government in Canada was not prepared actively to support her scheme financially, Groom was also told that 'no objections would be made to the admission of such persons into the country if they were protected by her'.[53] Further, as well as avoiding restrictions being imposed upon deaf and dumb migrants entering Canada by guaranteeing their financial independence through the Homesteader scheme, some government agents wrote positively about the settlers. For example, John Smith, an immigration agent, defended the scheme, writing:

> When I visited Manitoba I gave this subject [deaf mutes] considerable attention. And as Miss Groom has sent a number of people out there and as you say this class of immigration is not to be deprecated when considered with due regard to these unfortunate yet industrious and intelligent people for, to their credit be it said, there are no more honest safer hard working immigrants come out to this country.[54]

Another way of thinking about the potentially colonial implications of her idea to create a 'deaf colony' is to place it alongside that formulated some thirty years earlier by John Jacobus Flournoy (1808–79), the deaf son of a wealthy American slave-owner.[55] Flournoy, outraged at the discrimination that he faced as a deaf man, particularly by a law passed in Georgia reducing the status of deaf people to that of those with intellectual disabilities, wanted 'to secure the government and offices of a small territory or State, to the mute community'.[56] The scheme attracted much attention in the deaf community and was extensively debated in the deaf press for the rest of the century. Deaf people wrote both in support and in criticism of the deaf state, which some suggested might be called Deaf-Mutia or Gesturia.[57] Flournoy was also a virulent racist. His pamphlets, *A Reply to a Pamphlet Entitled, Bondage; A Moral Institution Sanctioned by the Scriptures and the Savior* and *An Essay on the origin, habits, and c. of the African race*, demonstrate a profound hatred of African Americans.[58] But the scheme, of course, if carried out, would also have displaced Native American people. While Groom never mentioned Flournoy's scheme, and certainly never expressed the vitriolic racism of Flournoy, comparing the schemes shows us how disability-based activism not only could coexist within imperial frameworks but could actively condone racist or colonialist agendas.

Analysis and conclusion

Positing any similarity between the lives of Kitto, Tait and Groom is difficult. They had profoundly diverse experiences, including of deafness and imperialism. But this chapter has sought to think about what can be learned when we consider them collectively. What, if anything, can be learned from thinking of them as having led imperial lives? And how can this help us to understand the Victorians and disability?

What we know about all three of the people whom I have examined in this chapter is that they travelled to imperial places and, as such, had lives that were inflected by empire. As white British people they would have enjoyed a certain amount of privilege in these imperial spaces, regardless of their disability. This is not to say that they necessarily endorsed imperialist values or that they did not also experience discrimination and marginalisation on account of their deafness. As I have stated earlier in this chapter, the purpose of my argument is not to condemn Kitto, Tait and Groom as 'bad apples' or as 'deaf imperialists' but, rather, to use their lives to think about what it meant that the Victorians were at the heart of a global empire.

One conclusion that can be drawn from looking at Kitto, Tait and Groom together is that empire was not something that affected only upper- or middle-class people; it was also experienced by people from working-class and, in Kitto's case, impoverished backgrounds. In his 2004 study, *The Absent-Minded Imperialists*, historian Bernard Porter argued that many working-class people were oblivious to the very existence of empire.[59] I disagree. Instead, I would argue that the lives of British people were inflected by empire, whether or not it was consciously registered as such. And further, that recognising these inflections is key if the British are to overcome what has been described as their 'historical amnesia' towards empire, which, among other things, has rendered many people oblivious to the destructive legacies of British imperialism, both in Britain and internationally, today. But what we can draw from Porter's argument is that going to places of empire did not necessarily mean that a person reflected on this, or engaged with an imperial ideology. None of the records of the three case studies that I have examined shows any active engagement with the concept of empire, or comments on Canada and Malta being part of the British Empire. Empire was simply something that existed, part of the backdrop of everyday life and the opportunities that were available to these three people.

We can conclude that, although there may be analogies drawn between being colonised and being disabled, these were not the same thing. Nor was the relationship between race and disability. Tait and Groom were able to use land in Canada precisely because they were not First Nations People, but were white British settlers. Kitto, meanwhile, was able to use his white privilege to his advantage in the Baghdad marketplace where his use of English, however impaired, gave him an elevated social status.

Another thing we can learn is that deafness was experienced and managed very differently by different people. While Kitto 'abominated sign language', both Groom and Tait were, to varying extents, sign language users. While Kitto distanced himself from other deaf people, both Groom and Tait sought them out, and found their deafness, in order to create bonds of connection in unexpected places. While all three were literate to some degree, their facility with written English varied, and this too would have shaped their lives. They also had differing degrees of connection with hearing people in the wider community; Groom cooperated with hearing philanthropists, while, particularly in his early life, Kitto found conversation with hearing people painful and tedious.

In sum, the three case studies of John Kitto, George Tait and Jane Groom that I have discussed in this chapter can be used to think about the complicated relationship between disability, race and colonialism. I have argued that colonialism played a part in the lives of each of these individuals, who, at least in some ways, were aligned with the coloniser. The early histories of disability in Britain have focused on recovering the lives of deaf and disabled people who have experienced and resisted various forms of disempowerment, particularly those of former residents of the schools and institutions that have proved so controversial. But reframing this work in a colonial context reminds us that such processes of disenfranchisement and exclusion were part of a wider shift in the constitution of a normative subject.

It also raises potentially uneasy questions about the ways in which people with disabilities, including deaf people, could occupy the position of an oppressor group as well as a group that has been repressed. Other examples might have been chosen to make this point more starkly. The partially deaf Francis Baring (1740–1810), for example, earned huge amounts of money from the transatlantic slave trade, and for some years directed the East India Company as it sought to exploit the Indian subcontinent.[60] Francis Humberstone Mackenzie (1754–1815) was also deaf and was involved in slavery, as well as being Governor of Barbados from 1800 to 1806.[61] But what I have intended to do here is not to blame Kitto, Tait or Groom for being part of this global system, but to argue that to understand the lives of deaf and disabled Victorians we need to have an understanding of the wider colonial situation of which they were a part, and not assume that disabled people were always on the side of colonial resistance.

Notes

1   T. Szasz, *Psychiatric Slavery* (New York, NY: The Free Press, 1977).

2   K. Hirsch, 'From colonization to civil rights: people with disabilities and gainful employment', in P. D. Blanck (ed.), *Employment, Disability, and the Americans with Disabilities Act: Issues in Law, Public Policy, and Research* (Evanston, IL: Northwestern University Press, 2000), pp. 412–31.

3   G. Goggin and C. Newell, *Disability in Australia: Exposing a Social Apartheid* (Sydney: University of New South Wales Press, 2004).

4   L. Kriegel, 'Uncle Tom and Tiny Tim: some reflections on the cripple as Negro', *The American Scholar*, 38:3 (1969), 412–30.

5   H. Lane, *The Mask of Benevolence: Disabling the Deaf Community* (New York, NY: Vintage Books. 1993), p. 31.

6   For more on 'ableism' see, for example, F. K. Campbell, *Contours of Ableism: The Production of Disability and Abledness* (Basingstoke: Palgrave Macmillan, 2009).

7   E. Cleall, 'Orientalising deafness: race and disability in imperial Britain', *Social Identities*, 21:1 (2015), 22–36.

8   M. Sherry 'Postcolonizing disability', *Wagadu*, 4 (2007), 10–22.

9   C. Hall, and S. O. Rose (eds), *At Home with the Empire: Metropolitan Culture and the Imperial World* (Cambridge: Cambridge University Press, 2006).

10 For more information on John Kitto's life see E. Cleall, 'Producing and managing deviance in the disabled colonial self: John Kitto the deaf traveller', in W. Jackson and E. J. Manktelow (eds), *Subverting Empire: Deviance and Disorder in the British Colonial World* (Basingstoke: Palgrave Macmillan, 2015), pp. 126–45. See also E. Bar-Yosef, 'The "deaf traveller", the "blind traveller" and constructions of disability in nineteenth-century travel writing', *Victorian Review*, 35:2 (2009), 133–55; J. Eadie, *Life of John Kitto* (Edinburgh, 1886); and W. M. Thayer, *From Poor-House to Pulpit;*

or, The triumphs of the late Dr. John Kitto, from boyhood to manhood (Boston, MA, 1859).

11 J. Kitto, *The Lost Senses* (London, 1845), p. 19.

12 *Ibid.*, p. 20.

13 A. N. Porter, *Religion versus Empire: British Protestant Missionaries and Overseas Expansion, 1700–1914* (Manchester: Manchester University Press, 2004).

14 For two very different treatments of this debate see B. Stanley, *The Bible and the Flag: Protestant Missions and British Imperialism in the Nineteenth and Twentieth Centuries* (Leicester: Apollo, 1990), and I. Copland, 'Christianity as an arm of empire: the ambiguous case of India under the company, c. 1813–1858', *Historical Journal*, 4 (2006), 1025–54.

15 E. Cleall, *Missionary Discourses of Difference: Negotiating Otherness in the British Empire, c. 1800–1900* (Basingstoke: Palgrave Macmillan, 2012).

16 J. Cox, 'Were the Victorian nonconformists the worst imperialists of them all?', *Victorian Studies*, 46:2 (2004), 243–55.

17 For work on the way in which race and gender shaped missionary practice see: C. Hall, *Civilising Subjects: Metropole and Colony in the English Imagination, 1830–1867* (Cambridge: Polity Press, 2002); C. Hall, 'Missionary stories: gender and ethnicity in England in the 1830s and 1840s', *White, Male and Middle Class: Explorations in Feminism and History* (Cambridge: Polity Press, 1995), pp. 205–55.

18 Cleall, *Missionary Discourses of Difference*, pp. 80–1.

19 R. Seton, '"Open doors for female labourers": women candidates of the London Missionary Society, 1875–1914', in R. Bickers and R. Seton, *Missionary Encounters: Sources and Issues* (Richmond: Curzon, 1996), pp. 63–4.

20 J. Kitto, 'Diary', in J. E. Ryland (ed.), *Memoir of John Kitto DD, chiefly compiled from his letters and journals* (New York, NY, 1856), p. 138.

21 J. Kitto to Mr Burnard (13 November 1827), Malta, reproduced in Ryland, *Memoir*, p. 255.

22 M. Dumper and B. E. Stanley, *Cities of the Middle East and North Africa: A Historical Encyclopedia* (Oxford: ABC-CLIO, 2007), p. 59.

23 Cleall, 'Producing and managing deviance'.

24 Kitto, *Lost Senses*, p. 118.

25 *Ibid.*, p. 100 (emphasis in original).

26 Cleall, 'Producing and managing deviance'.

27 J. Kitto to Mr Burnard (25 October 1830), Baghdad, reproduced in Ryland, *Memoir*, p. 375.

28 'The deaf traveller, 3', in *Penny Magazine*, 1833, 336.

29 'The deaf traveller, 5', in *Penny Magazine*, 1833, 407.

30 Cleall, 'Producing and managing deviance', p. 139.

31 For a more in-depth discussion of Tait's life see: E. Cleall, 'Deaf connections and global conversations: deafness and education in and beyond the British Empire, ca. 1800–1900', *Journal of Colonialism and Colonial History*, 16:1 (2015), n.p.

32 T. M. Devine, *To the Ends of the Earth: Scotland's Global Diaspora, 1750–2010* (London: Allen Lane, 2011); M. Harper and S. Constantine, *Migration and Empire* (Oxford: Oxford University Press, 2010).

33 G. Tait, *Autobiography of George Tait, A Deaf Mute* (Halifax, Nova Scotia, 1878), p. 4.

34 Cleall, 'Deaf connections'.

35 National Library of Scotland, Acc. 11896, Donaldson's Hospital, 'Applications for admission, 1810–1969', p. 272, 1861–74.

36 See Cleall, 'Deaf connections'.

37 Tait, *Autobiography*, p. 6.

38 *Ibid.*, p. 8.

39 *Ibid.*, p. 14.

40 Cleall, 'Deaf connections'.

41 L. Veracini, *Settler Colonialism: A Theoretical Overview* (Basingstoke: Palgrave Macmillan, 2010).

42 My thanks to Norma McGilp for sharing with me Jane Groom's death certificate, which has allowed me to accurately record the date of her death. For a more in-depth discussion of Jane Groom's life see: E. Cleall, 'Jane Groom and the deaf colonists: empire, emigration and the agency of disabled people in the late nineteenth-century British Empire', *History Workshop Journal*, 81:1 (2016), 39–61.

43 P. Ladd, *Understanding Deaf Culture: In Search of Deafhood* (Clevedon: Multilingual Matters, 2003), pp. 46–7.

44 'Jane Groom' (1881), census return for St John Hackney, Sub-district, West Hackney [online]. The National Archives: 296 folio 32 p. 26, Ancestry (2013). Available from: www.ancestry.co.uk, accessed 6 February 2013.

45 J. Branson and D. Miller, *Damned for Their Difference: The Cultural Construction of Deaf People as Disabled* (Washington, DC: Gallaudet University Press, 2002), pp. 154–5.

46 H. H., *A Future for the Deaf and Dumb in the Canadian North-West: Being an account of a first attempt at colonisation in the Canadian North-West* (London, 1884), p. 13.

47 H. H., *An Evangelist Among the Deaf and Dumb* (London, 1884), p. 6.

48 Cleall, 'Jane Groom and the deaf colonists'.

49 H. H., *An Evangelist*, p. 6.

50 P. Buckner, 'Tupper, Sir Charles', in *Dictionary of Canadian Biography*, available online at www.biographi.ca/009004–119.01-e.php?&id_nbr=7747.

51 National Canadian Archives (hereafter NCA), 1884/12/24, File FG17 427, Sir Charles Tupper, London, England.

52 H. H., *An Evangelist*, p. 7.

53 Memo to the Hon. John Carling, Minister of Agriculture, 5 Jan. 1891. For more information on entry being refused to prospective immigrants on the grounds of their disability see R. Hanes, 'None is still too many: an historical exploration of Canadian immigration legislation as it pertains to people with disabilities', *Developmental Disabilities Bulletin*, 37 (2009), 91–126; E. Chadha, '"Mentally defectives"

not welcome: mental disability in Canadian immigration law, 1859–1927', *Disability Studies Quarterly*, 28:1 (2008), n.p.; B. Roberts, 'Doctors and the deports: the role of the medical profession in Canadian deportation, 1900–20', *Canadian Ethnic Studies*, 13:3 (1986), 17–36; R. Menzies, 'Governing mentalities: the deportation of "insane" and "feebleminded" immigrants out of British Columbia from Confederation to World War II', *Canadian Journal of Law and Society, 13 (1998)*, 135–73.

54   NCA, RG17, 536, 'Letter from Mr John Smith [immigration agent] of Hamilton, Ontario, 21 May 1887 addressed to Mr Lowe'.

55   For more information on Flournoy see H. Joyner, *From Pity to Pride: Growing Up Deaf in the Old South* (Washington, DC: Gallaudet University Press, 2004), pp. 107–19.

56   J. J. Flournoy (1856) quoted in C. Krentz, *A Mighty Change: An Anthology of Deaf American Writing, 1816–1864* (Washington, DC: Gallaudet University Press, 2000), p. 165.

57   A selection of writings both for and against the deaf state is published in Krentz, *A Mighty Change*, pp. 161–211.

58   J. J. Flournoy *A Reply to a Pamphlet Entitled, Bondage; A Moral Institution Sanctioned by the Scriptures and the Savior* and *An Essay on the origin, habits, and c. of the African race* (1835). Other pamphlets highlighting his racist attitudes include 'A speech on our Indian relations and international policies: Elicited by the Seminole war' (1836).

59   B. Porter, *The Absent-minded Imperialists: Empire, Society and Culture in Britain* (Oxford: Oxford University Press, 2004), pp. 1–25. See also B. Porter, 'Empire, what Empire? Or why 80 per cent of early and mid-Victorians were deliberately kept in ignorance of it', *Victorian Studies*, 46:2 (2004), 256–63.

60   L. Davies, 'Sir Francis Baring, the deaf banker', *British Deaf History Society: Deaf History Journal*, 15:4 (2012), 14–16.

61   P. Jackson, 'Francis Humberstone Mackenzie', in P. Jackson and R. Lee (eds), *Deaf Lives: Deaf People in History* (Middlesex: Deaf History Society, 2001).

3

DISABLING THE AUTHOR IN MID-VICTORIAN REALIST FICTION: CASE STUDIES OF GEORGE ELIOT AND HARRIET MARTINEAU

Deborah M. Fratz

In literary studies George Eliot (1819–80) is often identified as the most ardent proponent of realism. Historical discussions of realism frequently invoke her letters, her novels and her review of two works by German ethnographer W. H. Riehl (1823–97). Today we read 'The Natural History of German Life' as a kind of manifesto for realist fiction. Eliot famously states that 'the greatest benefit we owe to the artist, whether painter, poet, or novelist, is the extension of our sympathies', but she problematises those sympathies when they are invoked by sentimental or idealised depictions of ordinary life.[1] She deplores such depictions of working-class people in paintings and fiction, and asserts that 'the unreality of their representations is a grave evil'.[2] The arts must be informed with accurate portrayals of ordinary life: 'We want to be taught to feel', she writes, but 'not for the heroic artisan or the sentimental peasant'.[3] In praising Riehl's ethnography, Eliot advocates using concrete observations of social life in artistic productions. Her argument in this review, published by *The Westminster Review* in 1856, has a fascinating antecedent in the works of one of the most prolific writers of the Victorian era: Harriet Martineau (1802–76), an unmarried, middle-class author and traveller, who became almost entirely deaf by the age of eighteen.

Critics from many disciplines acknowledge how the social experience of deafness informed Martineau's theorisation of social observation, as outlined in her essay 'Letter to the Deaf', which appeared in *Tait's Edinburgh Magazine* in 1834. Her 1838 text, *How to Observe Morals and Manners*, describes the requisites and protocols for systematic social observation, which established Martineau as a kind of 'mother of sociology'. Martineau wrote widely, and, like

Eliot, she wrote one realist novel, *Deerbrook* (1838). Both authors extol the value of observing concrete social phenomena in order to increase understanding of social difference, and their similar handling of the subject is worth noting. From a disability studies perspective, my first goal is to draw attention to Martineau's understanding of disability as offering unique opportunities to make social observations.

Another similarity merits exploration: both writers authored realist novels featuring a central disabled character. Criticism addressing the use of disabled characters in Victorian fiction, such as Martha Stoddard Holmes's *Fictions of Affliction*, frequently acknowledges how such characters function by invoking feelings of sympathy, both within the narrative and in readers.[4] However, *Deerbrook*'s Maria Young and Philip Wakem in *The Mill on the Floss* (1860) reverse our expectations: rather than being the subjects of observation and sympathy, they operate as model observers, such as Martineau and Eliot describe. *Deerbrook*'s Maria Young particularly seems to reflect Martineau's prescriptions for social observation, and indeed, her 'post of observation' allows readers to observe the action of the novel as she does, as a social observer.[5]

However, when she shares her observations with other characters, internalised gender norms frustrate Maria's power to express her views. Similarly, while Philip's experience of social marginalisation shapes him into a keen observer with artistic ambitions, he voices his frustration with his power to express himself. Examining Martineau's and Eliot's disabled characters may establish that Maria Young and Philip Wakem, figured as sympathetic observers of their society, inhabit a narratorial position similar to that of their creators. While they sympathetically observe their societies, and even operate as moral mentors to other characters, their compromised powers of expression may dimly reflect Martineau's and Eliot's own frustrations with the realist mode. I rely exclusively on primary sources to establish a pattern for my hypothesis; more recent scholarship on realism and sympathy may productively enhance the possibility that disabled characters may reflect realism's limitations.

'A book well-nourished with specific facts'

Martineau's methodology for social observation undoubtedly arises from her experience of disability. Although she was a well-educated, middle-class woman, deafness prevented her from becoming a governess, as her sisters were. Instead, she turned to writing. The immense popularity of *Illustrations of Political Economy* (1834) confirmed her career as a writer and allowed her the confidence to expand the scope of her work to include travel writing, household advice and impassioned arguments for the abolition of slavery in America and for extending education for women. Despite genuine regret over her increasing deafness, Martineau sees opportunities even in her loss and, further, insists that the deaf must maintain social communication at all costs. In 'Letter to the Deaf', she addresses her 'fellow sufferers' – those who have become progressively deaf – by simultaneously acknowledging limitations 'as a plain matter of fact' and emphasising the possibilities that remain by asking: 'what must be given up, and what may be struggled for?'[6]

Even if excluded from conversation, the deaf may observe a rich array of social interactions. In one anecdote, a hostess asks Martineau how she manages to entertain herself when left out of the dinner conversation. She replies, 'I watch how you help the soup', as well as facial expressions and interactions among the servants.[7] Martineau insists that her limitation creates other opportunities:

> We are ... good perceivers in every way, and have ... rather that advantage over others in the power of abstract reasoning. This union of two kinds of power ... puts a considerable amount of accurate knowledge within easier reach of us than of most other people. We must never forget what a vast quantity we must forego, but neither must we lose sight of whatever is peculiarly within our power.[8]

Exclusion from social exchanges allows deaf people to cultivate the qualities of good sociologists: to observe others with a degree of distance and to have the time to contemplate what has been observed. What Martineau calls 'abstract reasoning' lays the foundation for a philosophy of social observation that depends on cultivated sympathy for the subjects of enquiry. Martineau's advice in 'Letter to the Deaf' corresponds to the theory and practice of social observation described in *How to Observe Morals and Manners*. Her reflections on her experience as a deaf woman inspired her theories of social observation.

How to Observe Morals and Manners established Martineau as a kind of proto-sociologist. The observational powers Martineau attributes to the deaf, and, by extension, to others who inhabit social margins, correspond to those cultivated by the traveller in *How to Observe Morals and Manners*. In this text limitations also have value. Just as the deaf must accept 'what must be given up', the social observer limits the scope of enquiry, choosing to observe specific aspects of a society. Similarly, Martineau advises making concrete, visible phenomena the primary source of information. She claims that because the 'discourse of persons' tends to represent an individual's views rather than social institutions, it should be understood only as 'commentary' on what the traveller has independently observed.[9] Her term 'manners' broadly refers to the observable social practices of a culture, such as 'architectural remains, epitaphs, civic registers, national music' – those things that allow the observer to see 'manifestations of the common mind.'[10] Again, we may easily see how Martineau acquired a sense of this practice as a deaf woman: unable to enter conversations, her primary source of information was what she may observe.

Similarly, Eliot took great interest in the methods of social observation, as evidenced in 'The Natural History of German Life'. Her praise of W. H. Riehl's ethnographic survey of peasant life in rural Germany has a distinct agenda. She writes, 'What we are desiring for ourselves has been in some degree done for the Germans by Riehl', and, in drawing attention to his text, she hopes that British readers will see 'a model for some future or actual student of our own people': someone of 'sufficient moral and intellectual breadth', who 'would devote himself to studying the natural history of our social classes' by making first-hand observation of 'local conditions', 'maxims and habits' and 'the interaction of the various classes on each other'.[11] A collection of such observations, 'a book well-nourished with specific facts', would be 'a valuable aid to the social and political reformer'.[12] Indeed, Eliot admires Riehl for doing precisely what Martineau prescribes in *How to Observe Morals and Manners*. Thus, both authors share a deep investment in observing the concrete objects and activities of ordinary life as signs of social values.

Eliot's agenda differs from Martineau's. While the latter prescribes observation to serve science – albeit an early form of the discipline that will become social science – the novelist focuses on art. Eliot links the necessity of accurate observations with art, and art with sympathy: 'Art is the nearest thing to life; it is a mode of amplifying experience and extending our contact with our fellow-men beyond the bounds of our personal lot.'[13] For art to actually *be* the nearest thing to life, it must rely on first-hand observations of life; the artist must not filter what he sees through inherited misconceptions or generalisations, and specifically, Eliot warns against the mistake which she sees in novelists: 'they transfer their own feelings to ploughmen and woodcutters, and give them both joys and sorrows of which they know nothing.'[14] Despite her arguments for objectivity, Eliot does not abolish 'feelings' from the production or reception of literature, but insists that author–observers self-consciously separate their own affect from what they observe in others. If art is effective and readers experience the 'extension of our sympathies', those sympathies must be for the ploughman and woodcutter as they truly are.[15]

For Martineau, sympathy is the means and end of social observation. Much of *How to Observe Morals and Manners* focuses on understanding practices and institutions by first acknowledging that all human activity arises out of what Martineau perceived as the universal desire to pursue happiness and social good. Failing to observe with an open mind limits access to good information and the ability to assess it meaningfully. If an observer judges others by his own cultural values, 'he will not be admitted with freedom into the retirements of domestic life', which is where the best information may be found.[16] The 'discourse of persons' will be equally limited, as 'people will talk to him of the things they care least about, instead of seeking his sympathy about the affairs which are deepest in their hearts.[17] If an observer is 'full of sympathy, everything he sees will be instructive, and the most important matters will be the most clearly revealed.[18]

Martineau's social observer, like the one described by Eliot, begins with sympathy and, having acquired information, may then expand sympathy in others who read it. Accurately presenting social information has a moral imperative, as Martineau writes, 'what work on earth is more serious than this …? Every true report is a great good; every untrue report is a great mischief.[19] Eliot asserts the same thing twenty years later: sympathy must be formed for people as they actually are.

The disabled characters in *Deerbrook* and *The Mill on the Floss* share qualities with their realist authors in how they observe, assess, sympathise and mentor. Martineau's lamed governess, Maria Young, has a narrator's authority, and Eliot's Philip Wakem develops artistic abilities through careful observation. In the same way that authors are removed from their narratives, the characters' social exclusion allows them to assess what they observe with what Martineau calls 'the power of abstract reasoning.[20] Their contemplative natures allow Maria and Philip to suffer the emotional trauma of unrequited love yet generously assess the complex relationships between their rivals and lovers. The sympathy and mentorship they extend to central characters are important. For both Maria and Philip, their disabled subject position allows them to cultivate powers of observation and sympathy that grant them moral authority that may benefit others. But when Martineau and Eliot end their realist novels by isolating these remarkable characters, readers tend to see Maria and Philip as pitiable, an appalling revocation of their agency. What these disabled characters achieve in these novels, with their powers to observe, sympathise and provide moral guidance, is similar to what authors do. They observe social interactions and institutions and offer readers moral guidance. However, the conflicts which the disabled characters face – frustrated expression and the loss of opportunity to share their enlightened views – might also reflect the anxieties of their authors.

Martineau's Maria Young: in a post of observation

Although Maria shares characteristics with her creator, reading this character as a stand-in for Martineau is not the objective here. Martineau certainly used her own experience as an educated, unmarried, disabled woman to imagine a narrative about a young woman relying on her own capacities and, far from regretting what most Victorians would see as disadvantages, Martineau capitalised on these qualities. Maria likewise articulates her limitations as opportunities. When her lameness prevents her from flower gathering with friends, she muses,

> It is a luxury ... for one who cannot move about to sit here and look abroad. ... To overlook people, – to watch them acting unconsciously, and speculate for them! ... why should I not watch for others? Every situation has its privileges and its obligations. – What is it to be alone, and to be let alone, as I am? It is to be put into a post of observation on others: but the knowledge so gained is anything but a good if it stops at mere knowledge, – if it does not make me feel and act.[21]

From the standpoint of disability studies, we see a fascinating reversal of social expectations. In 'Letter to the Deaf', as well as in *Deerbrook*, the disabled are empowered in several ways: by making social exclusion an opportunity to observe, and those observations the basis of tolerance, the disabled subject position evolves from a passive object of sympathy to a perceptive, active and sympathetic observer of society. Far from being a victim of her circumstances, Maria seizes opportunities and recognises how her observations potentially serve others.

Maria uses her power to 'feel and act' when she becomes a kind of mentor to Margaret Ibbotson, one of two orphaned sisters whose struggles with courtship and marriage inform the novel's major plot threads.[22] However, when Maria observes the rules of romantic love she does not fully articulate what she observes. Maria and Margaret have much in common. Maria was also orphaned, after a carriage accident left her lame and her father dead, and both women are in love with the same man. Maria's disabling injury excludes her from the marriage market, requiring her to support herself as a governess. Her former beau turns his attentions to Margaret, but without declaring himself, thus creating anxiety for both women. Margaret worries that her love is not returned, and Maria suffers from unrequited love, a vow of silence and life-long social instability.

In a carefully worded conversation, Maria neither directly states that she sees that Margaret is in love nor admits that she loves the same man. She alludes to the source of Margaret's anxiety, intimates that she has suffered the same way and explains the feminine necessity of hiding romantic feelings. While love and death both traumatise, mourning death at least invites the comfort of others: 'all that we can conceive to happen in death ... happens in love, with the additional burden of fearful secrecy'.[23] If a Victorian woman cannot be certain that her love is returned, duty 'calls upon her to endure, silently and alone'.[24] However hyperbolic this language, it accurately describes the restraint expected from Victorian women. This imposed silence smothers Maria's hopes to use her knowledge for a greater good.

Maria's frustration lies in that 'fearful secrecy' and silence. However accurate her observations, and however deeply informed her sympathy may be, secrecy requires repressing what she longs to say. Like her creator, Maria tries to turn even this burden into an opportunity by asserting, 'there is not on earth a being stronger than a woman in the concealment of her love. ... How noble is such power of self-restraint!'[25] Vindicating the silence of a character who makes excellent observations signals a conflict. On the one hand, to 'speculate' on the lives of others and to 'feel and act' is empowering. Maria's sympathetic observations of Margaret comfort both of them and, as the narrative continues, readers see how Margaret's traumatic experience of courtship is alleviated by Maria's sympathy and mentorship. On the other hand, when gender norms prohibit describing her observations, her power diminishes. Maria may speak only to another woman facing the same issues, and thus her observations have limited value; further, what she can actually say is restricted. The potential for increasing sympathy for those on the margins of society is truncated by stifled expression. Maria may be 'clear-sighted, [and] ready to help' with the wisdom gained through sympathetic observation, but socially sanctioned silence will be no help at all.[26]

By the end of the work, we sense Martineau's conflicted interests in writing a realist novel. Maria's extraordinary agency declines after Margaret marries. Losing her confidante, she loses one of the few opportunities to help someone with her sympathetic observations. Margaret grimly assesses her friend's situation: 'you are infirm and suffering in body, poor, solitary, living by toil, without love, without prospect'.[27] Readers understandably pity her, but Martineau would find this distasteful. The author understood women's limited economic options, and that women like Maria – and herself – are rare. Yet, in *Deerbrook* no one can imagine good options for Maria; not Margaret, not Maria, nor Martineau herself. A realist novel about the lives of middle-class Victorian women inevitably focuses on marriage – some women are saved while others are doomed without it. Realism, with its accurate portrayal of society, conflicts with Martineau's ambitions – to help readers understand their society in order to improve it.

Martineau's subsequent fiction, such as her historical romance novel about Touissant L'Ouverture, *The Hour and the Man* (1839), avoided realist treatment. *Forest and Game Law Tales* (1845–46) returns to the same fable-like form she used in *Illustrations of Political Economy* (1832), and most of her later writing is devoted to history and politics. The very practice she praises – the accurate

representation of the operations of society – frustrates her attempts to write
didactically in the realist mode.

Eliot's Philip Wakem: studying expression

Eliot's depiction of Philip Wakem follows a similar trajectory, though artistic
ambitions shape his conflict differently. When Tom Tulliver meets Philip at
school, the scene links Philip's artistic talent with his disability. After watching
Philip draw, Tom harbours 'a puzzled suspicion that Philip's crooked back might
be the source of remarkable faculties.'[28] Sensitive to how a new student will
react to his hunched back, Philip hides his discomfort by taking up his drawing
pencil. In words reminiscent of Martineau's, he states: 'You've only to look well
at things, and draw them over and over again. What you do wrong once, you
can alter the next time.'[29] The social observer must 'look well at things', and the
repetition of drawing parallels the process of contemplation of observed
phenomena. Altering what was done 'wrong' suggests that contemplation compels
someone like Philip (or Martineau, or Eliot) to carefully represent what has
been observed. Tom's naïve essentialisation of Philip's disability, linking physical
difference with an unusual talent, mirrors Victorian attitudes towards physical
difference, but with Martineau's perspectives we can see how the social experience
of disability might cultivate the capacity to 'look well at things', as Philip does.

   Careful observation characterises Philip's relationship with Maggie Tulliver.
When Maggie visits Tom at school, her intellectual curiosity and uninhibited
affection impress Philip so deeply that he preserves his memory of her in a
painted miniature. Years later, her portrait testifies to Philip's observational
powers and artistic temperament. Meeting her again, he tells Maggie, 'I watched
a long while ... near your house to see if you would come out, but you never
came. Then I watched again to-day, and when I saw the way you took, I kept
you in sight.'[30] Philip's 'seeing' and 'watching' facilitates their reunion, in which
he offers her books to inspire her to become the 'brilliant woman, – all wit and
bright imagination', that he knows she can be.[31] Philip's powers of observation
and sympathy, acquired through the social experience of disability, make him
uniquely able to recognise her intellect, sensitivity and depth of feeling. In many
ways, Philip is crucial to Maggie's moral development. When Maggie faces the
novel's central crisis, her self-awareness and powers of sympathy underpin a
sophisticated ethical consciousness that develops through her relationship with
Philip.

   Philip has personal interest in Maggie's expansion. One of the few people
to show him affection, she may be the only woman willing to marry him. Just
as Maria Young's lameness removed her from the marriage market in *Deerbrook*,

Philip's physical difference reduces the likelihood of sexual love and marriage – desires that Eliot treats with unsentimental candour. Without physical prowess, townspeople say, Philip is 'no better than a girl', and while Maggie enjoys Philip's attention, sharing his interest in art and literature, she feels more pity than love for him.[32] He senses this, but nurtures hope on the barest traces of her affection. Maria Young's exclusion from the marriage market has more serious consequences – Philip's family wealth and his gender grant him more security – but, significantly, both characters experience unrequited love that will frustrate their powers of expression and weaken the agency they gain as social observers.

Eliot links Philip's frustrated artistic expression with his frustrated desire. Despite his excellent observations, Philip doubts his ability to express what he sees. He complains that he thinks 'of too many things, – sow all sorts of seeds, and get no great harvest from any one of them. I'm cursed with susceptibility in every direction, and effective faculty in none.'[33] Philip might have benefited by Martineau's suggestion to limit the scope of observation, but, more importantly, he voices his frustration with acting on his artistic impulses, in a manner similar to Maria Young's acknowledgment of the 'fearful secrecy' that limits her power to express her ideas. Philip suggests that he would accept artistic failure if Maggie loves him: 'nothing could make life worth the purchase-money of pain to [him], but some faculty' or 'a passion [that] answers as well as a faculty.'[34] Readers recognise Philip's intentions immediately – Maggie's love will reconcile him to his life – yet they also see Philip's failure to communicate this to Maggie, as she 'did not hear the last words', too absorbed as she was in her 'own discontent.'[35] Philip fails to win Maggie, and thus his purpose differs significantly from Martineau's and Eliot's. However, the proximity of his declared frustration with artistic expression and his concrete failure to express himself can reflect the questions posed here. What parallels can be established between a disabled character's powers of observation, sympathetic interpretation and frustrated expression and those same patterns in realist fiction?

Philip's powers of observation and sympathy reach their height in the last book of *The Mill on the Floss*, but he fails to use those powers effectively. He retreats from society when overpowered by emotion, and his absence and silence recall the same fate as Maria Young. Though they are separated by a long-standing legal feud between their families, Philip continues to watch Maggie and, more pointedly, her interactions with her cousin's undeclared fiancé, Stephen. Philip detects their mutual attraction before they acknowledge it themselves. His rivalry with Stephen is often presented in terms of observation: what Philip sees and how others see his watchful presence. Stephen notices Philip's intense scrutiny and asks if he is planning a portrait, to which Philip replies, 'I have been studying expression.'[36] Indeed, Philip's observations are so acute that he can see through

Stephen's feigned indifference to Maggie and, irritated by Stephen's rivalry and hypocrisy, he storms off.

This scene features Philip's acute perception and signals a flaw in his characterisation as a social observer. Fleeing society when emotionally overwhelmed violates Martineau's prescription for the deaf, as she writes that 'social communication must be kept up through all its pains, for the sake of our friends as well as for our own'.[37] When in society, Philip reads people well, and even sympathetically, but his self-imposed seclusion abolishes the agency he gains as an observer. He also fails to take advantage of his opportunities. He gains his father's consent to court Maggie, despite the animosity between their families, but fails to communicate this directly to Maggie: 'he shrank from that; but he had told everything to Lucy, with the hope that Maggie, being informed through her, might give him some encouraging sign'.[38] Whatever powers Philip has gained as an observer, he loses when he fails to communicate, placing him in a similar position to Maria Young.

Yet Philip's response to Maggie's moral crisis redeems him, revealing his utmost power of sympathy and expression. After an overnight boating trip with Stephen, Maggie returns to St Ogg's unmarried, thus demolishing her reputation. To marry Stephen would pain Lucy and Philip: 'I have caused sorrow already,' she tells Stephen, 'but I have never deliberately consented to it; I have never said, "They shall suffer, that I may have joy."'[39] Her self-sacrifice, ironically, figures her as a fallen woman, because no one in St Ogg's can comprehend her thinking – except Philip. His last letter illustrates his ability to see Maggie's situation for what it is rather than what it seems to be, and his dispassionate sympathy goes beyond forgiveness. He acknowledges his jealousy and grief, accepting such feelings as 'those terrible throes that love must suffer before it can be disembodied of selfish desire'.[40] Understanding Maggie is figured as an artistic production: 'I feel about you as the artist does about the scene over which his soul has brooded with love.'[41] Here, Philip expresses himself as an artist of profound compassion:

> You have been to my affections what light, what colour is to my eyes, what music is to the inward ear, you have raised a dim unrest into a vivid consciousness. The new life I have found in caring for [you] has transformed the spirit of rebellious murmuring into that willing endurance which is the birth of strong sympathy. … I even think sometimes that this gift of transferred life, which has come to me in loving you, may be a new power to me.[42]

Despite earlier complaints about artistic expression, this letter reveals remarkable eloquence and insights, and evidence that his artistic observations inspire so strong a sympathy that it moves him to 'that enlarged life which grows and grows by appropriating the life of others' – a phrase very like one of Eliot's best-known pronouncements: 'Art is the nearest thing to life; it is a mode of amplifying experience and extending our contact with our fellow-men beyond the bounds of our personal lot.'[43] Martineau would commend him for seeing his loss as a 'gift' and 'a new power'. Unlike Maria, Philip's powers of expression are, at this point, as strong as his powers of observation, and yet they will share a similar conclusion. Just as Maria loses her remarkable agency with Margaret's marriage, Philip loses his when Maggie dies.

Following the trajectory of Philip's development as an artist leads to a disheartening conclusion. He begins with a unique capacity for making careful observations and forming sympathetic interpretations; he articulates his desire to be an artist as well as his frustration with artistic expression; he foils his ambitions by deliberately fleeing social interaction and refusing to express himself, even to Maggie; and yet, when he suffers most, he shows a remarkable, expansive consciousness that directly arises from his social experience of disability. Yet, as the novel ends, he is reduced to life as a solitary visitor to Maggie's grave. The moral epiphany revealed in his letter is negated by his self-imposed isolation. Philip might have developed as an artist – perhaps as a writer – or he might have turned his powers of sympathy toward others. At the end of *The Mill on the Floss*, all of his potential is drained. When he is no longer a social observer, 'the birth of strong sympathy' suffers crib death.[44] His artistic capacity diminishes with the decline of these powers. He is even disembodied as a 'revisiting spirit', so the fact of his physical disability is negated as well, but not in any liberating sense.[45]

Conclusion

For both Maria and Philip their disabled subject position allows them to cultivate powers of observation and sympathy that grant them moral authority that may benefit others. But, when Martineau and Eliot end their realist novels by isolating these remarkable characters, readers tend to see Maria and Philip as pitiable, an appalling revocation of their agency. What these disabled characters achieve in these novels, with their powers to observe, sympathise and provide moral guidance, is similar to what authors do. They observe social interactions and institutions and offer readers moral guidance. However, the conflicts which the disabled characters face – frustrated expression and the loss of opportunity to share their enlightened views – might also reflect the anxieties of their authors.

I am suggesting that the problem might be the realist mode itself, and that the conflict can be reflected in the characterisation of disabled subjects. On the one hand, realism favours the accurate observation of society in order to cultivate sympathy for people as they actually are. On the other hand, presenting social phenomena in the realist mode creates conflicts with the author's own ideals. For Martineau, women ought to have options for economic support and personal development outside of marriage, but in *Deerbrook* they do not. For Eliot, personal suffering ought to lead to expanded sympathy that facilitates meaningful artistic expression and a capacity to share that sympathy and vision with others, but it does not. After *Deerbrook*, Martineau's writing steered away from realism, using her powers of social observation for other purposes. Eliot remains one of the exemplars of Victorian realism. She never gave it up, although she followed *The Mill on the Floss* with *Romola* (1862–63), which might be described as a historical romance. Establishing the authors' rejection of realism is not the point here. Instead, I wish to explore their frustrations with it, and to link that frustration with the presence of disabled characters.

Criticism on nineteenth-century realist fiction now accepts that even the most impassioned proponents of the realist mode were able to see its limitations. Historically, realism's reputation suffered under the rise of modernism, with its focus on the splintering effects of language and disrupted forms. Realism was viewed as smugly invested in empirical representations which facilitated the unravelling of a unified truth that could be seen with careful observation. Yet George Levine argues that realism was 'not a solidly self-satisfied vision based in a misguided objectivity and faith in representation, but a highly self-conscious attempt to explore or create a new reality. Its massive self-confidence implied a radical doubt, its strategies of truth telling, a profound self-consciousness.'[46] The works of Martineau and Eliot seem to reflect that self-consciousness and desire to 'create a new reality' in their disabled characters who also reveal 'a radical doubt'.[47] In both realist novels, the authors do not depict 'a new reality' so much as show the consequences of social institutions as they are. In *Deerbrook* women must suffer for love and keep silent; in *The Mill on the Floss* a blameless woman will endure a bad reputation because her community has judged her according to appearances rather than a complicated truth. In both novels the disabled are pushed to the margins and silenced. Through the inclusion of disabled characters, operating somewhat like their authors, the radical doubt that Levine identifies has a more concrete representation.

Returning to the non-literary texts reveals their common interest in using accurate social observations to inform the public. Martineau encourages her observer 'to be useful rather than shining; to be the servant rather than the lord of science, a friend to the home-stayers rather than their dictator.'[48] Eliot's formulation is more concrete. Those books 'well-nourished with specific facts' can train the artist in a way of seeing; the artist's work may then present 'a picture of human life [that] surprises even the trivial and the selfish into that attention to what is a part from themselves which may be called the raw material of moral sentiment'.[49] Whether a work of social science, like Riehl's, or a novel, like Eliot's, 'a book well-nourished with specific facts' can 'be a valuable aid to the social and political reformer'.[50] Both Martineau and Eliot anticipate that the reader's insights and sympathies, acquired through the reading experience, move outward in an expanded understanding of others. What the reader felt for Maria and Margaret or Maggie and Philip will inform how the reader feels about meeting their counterparts in real life.

Rebecca Mitchell offers a valuable counterpoint. While maintaining that 'novels teach us how to empathise', her argument revises assumptions about how empathy develops.[51] Mitchell distinguishes between knowing 'the other' in a work of art and knowing 'the other' in real life. Only in art is another person knowable. Like Levine, Mitchell asserts that realist authors 'recognize the limitations of their depictions':

> The author cannot make her characters something other than they are; the painter cannot represent every mystery hidden in his subjects. Rather than being a flaw in the realist doctrine, these limits attest to the realities of life in community with others. ... Novels and paintings may be utterly knowable, but those they depict ... cannot be completely understood by others within the works.[52]

When novels reveal how characters fail to truly 'know' each other, that very failure reflects real life. We can know characters in art, but will never know one another in the same way. Mitchell suggests that this is in fact realism's purpose: to highlight the unknowable nature of another human being – which hardly seems the foundation for creating the sympathetic expansion Eliot hopes for. Mitchell's assessment is not dire – in the examples she chooses, 'in the very movement toward an appreciation for alterity are the seeds of mutuality'.[53] Her readings show the positive potential of recognising difference, and that achieving empathy with another might not be the goal, so much as aspiring towards that recognition. In this chapter, I have sought to show a similar kind of aspiration in those works and characters in which the aspiration is frustrated.

Victorian literature abounds with disabled characters, and some of them follow the pattern I describe here. In Charles Dickens' *Our Mutual Friend* (1864–55), Jenny Wren can see multiple masculine threats to her dear friend, but she never directly warns Lizzie about them.[54] In Elizabeth Gaskell's *Ruth* (1853), Thurstan Benson's sensitivity and compassion allow him to see Ruth's potential for atonement, but self-imposed silence keeps him from speaking the truth on her behalf.[55] The presence of these disabled characters in realist fiction invites the comparison between their positions as observers, narrators and artists and the position of their authors. By granting disabled characters some of the same qualities as realist authors, realist novelists might be representing their frustration with the realist mode. Further research in the acknowledged limitations of realism and in the extraordinary agency of disabled characters might productively explore a significant pattern in the dominant literary form of the Victorian era.

Notes

1 G. Eliot, 'The natural history of German life', in N. Sheppard (ed.), *The Essays of George Eliot* (Whitefish, MT: Kessinger Publishing, 2010), p. 141.
2 *Ibid.*
3 *Ibid.*
4 M. S. Holmes, *Fictions of Affliction: Physical Disability in Victorian Culture* (Ann Arbor, MI: University of Michigan Press, 2004).
5 H. Martineau, *Deerbrook* (1838).
6 H. Martineau, 'Letter to the Deaf', *Tait's Edinburgh Magazine* (1834).
7 *Ibid.*
8 *Ibid.*
9 H. Martineau, *How to Observe Morals and Manners* (1838), p. 63.
10 *Ibid.*, p. 64.
11 Eliot, 'The natural history of German life', p. 148.
12 *Ibid.*
13 *Ibid.*, p. 146.
14 *Ibid.*, p. 156.
15 *Ibid.*, p. 145.
16 Martineau, *How to Observe*, p. 44.
17 *Ibid.*
18 *Ibid.*, p. 48.
19 *Ibid.*, p. 17.
20 Martineau, 'Letter to the Deaf'.
21 Martineau, *Deerbrook*.
22 *Ibid.*
23 *Ibid.*
24 *Ibid.*
25 *Ibid.*
26 *Ibid.*
27 *Ibid.*
28 G. Eliot, *The Mill on the Floss* (1860).
29 *Ibid.*
30 *Ibid.*
31 *Ibid.*
32 *Ibid.*
33 *Ibid.*

34 *Ibid.*
35 *Ibid.*
36 *Ibid.*
37 Martineau, 'Letter to the Deaf'.
38 Eliot, *The Mill on the Floss.*
39 *Ibid.*
40 *Ibid.*
41 *Ibid.*
42 *Ibid.*
43 *Ibid.*; Eliot, 'The natural history of German life', p. 146.
44 Eliot, *The Mill on the Floss.*
45 *Ibid.*
46 G. Levine, *The Realistic Imagination: English Fiction from Frankenstein to Lady Chatterley* (Chicago, IL: University of Chicago Press, 1981), pp. 19–20.
47 *Ibid.*, p. 20.
48 Martineau, *How to Observe*, p. 10.
49 Eliot, 'The natural history of German life', pp. 148, 145.
50 *Ibid.*, p. 145.
51 R. N. Mitchell, *Victorian Lessons on Empathy and Difference* (Columbus, OH: Ohio State University Press, 2011), p. x.
52 *Ibid.*, p. 26.
53 *Ibid.*
54 C. Dickens, *Our Mutual Friend* (1864–65).
55 E. Gaskell, *Ruth* (1853).

Part II

INTERVENTIONS

4

MEDICALISING DEAFNESS IN VICTORIAN LONDON: THE ROYAL EAR HOSPITAL, 1816–1900

Jaipreet Virdi

A few steps from the vibrant and convivial atmosphere of London's Soho Square stands a plain, four-storey brick house on Carlisle Street where, in 1816, aural surgeon John Harrison Curtis (1776–1860) first opened the doors of the Royal Dispensary for Diseases of the Ear (RDDE). Believing that medical practitioners frequently overlooked aural ailments as incidental objects to other diseases, Curtis presented the dispensary as an approach for addressing a crucial social need, namely, the 'problem of deafness': how to best assimilate deaf persons into hearing society. Later renamed the Royal Ear Hospital, the institution would become a 'world-focusing point for the most advanced knowledge' of ear diseases, a place for ground-breaking research and innovative treatment.[1] It transformed medical and social conceptions about the curability of deafness by providing specialised care and undermining the proliferation of advertised nostrums and emetics that too often were useless or worsened the affliction.[2] In this transformation, the RDDE would legitimise the medical infrastructure that enabled nineteenth-century aural specialists – also known as 'aurists' – to exert their authority over deaf bodies.

The Victorian age was a period when deafness became pathologised and constructed as a deviation from the human norm. Deafness, and disability more broadly, Victorians believed, was a personal tragedy that required extensive medical intervention to 'overcome' bodily limitations, replacing earlier religious and moral imperatives that cast blame on the individual for their failings. While the early nineteenth century saw the basis laid of what would become Deaf culture, with a separate identity unified by sign language, by the 1870s, broader eugenic debates on the nature of man led to increased cultural emphasis on self-presentation and social mobility.[3] This shift reflected new cultural concerns about the disabled body in Victorian England, and the role of deaf persons as functioning, employed and fulfilled citizens.[4]

Deafness, then, became a condition to be treated and cured, placed exclusively in the domain of medical experts.[5] Part of the shift was grounded in oralist demands for the deaf to be 'hearing-minded': to seek out 'cures' for their afflictions, make use of assistive devices or, at the very least, 'pass' as hearing.[6] Guided by new knowledge in the physiology, anatomy and diseases of the ear – and a greater incidence of successful treatments – aurists stressed that deafness *could* be curable if only it was properly assessed by a qualified practitioner.

This chapter argues that the shift towards a more medicalised construction of deafness can be examined through the RDDE and the approaches to treatment offered during the course of its history. Within a broader history of deafness, the RDDE signified a new perception of hearing impairment, solidifying the notion that deafness was a medical, rather than educational or social, responsibility.[7] This did not mean that Curtis, or other aurists at the time, disregarded claims for social reform in conjunction with their medical work. Nor did it mean that the medical image displaced the social one.[8] Rather than creating strict demarcation between the 'medical' and 'social' models of disability, or undermining the richness of Deaf culture, examining the history of medical treatments for hearing loss and how aurists attempted to assert their authority over deaf bodies can provide us with a more nuanced picture of the history of deafness. Indeed, as Julie Anderson and Beth Linker have argued, the role of medicine and medical developments is interwoven within disability history.[9] As Coreen McGuire has stressed, to dismiss medicine is tantamount to ignoring the full experiences of deaf persons in history.[10]

As historians have shown, the value of dispensaries and specialised hospitals relied upon how they were able to address social needs.[11] As charitable institutions, they played a vital role in shaping the power and positions of medical specialists, providing opportunities for self-interest and routes 'to power, prestige, and wealth', as noted by Lindsay Granshaw.[12] Such institutions also relied heavily upon the reputations of their founders and directors, a dependency that could at times threaten the respectability of their social agenda. This chapter begins with an overview of Curtis's motivations for establishing the RDDE and the pre-1840s trend of aurists to boast curability for all cases of deafness – even though some cautiously argued that cases of congenital or 'nervous' deafness were beyond the purview of the surgeon. As Jennifer Esmail asserts, the growth of aural surgery was one of the varied ways in which British culture intervened in the issue of deafness.[13] By next turning to the expansion and then the eventual relocation of the RDDE after the 1840s, this chapter contextualises how aurists strove to pathologise hearing loss through individual treatment.

The founding years: 1816–36

When John Harrison Curtis first opened the doors of his dispensary, his practice was challenged by his competitors, notably the more-established aurists John Stevenson (1778–1844) and William Maule (1775–1851), Maule being the official aurist to the royal family. They insisted that Curtis's training as a dispenser in the Royal Navy did not constitute proper medical qualifications, and that his entrepreneurial spirit was a disgrace to the profession.[14] However, tales of Curtis's successful treatments drew patients to his door. His restoration of hearing in a sixty-year-old patient even attracted the attention of the Prince Regent, who appointed Curtis 'Aurist-to-his-Person' in 1817 and presented royal patronage to the dispensary.[15]

Renamed the Royal Dispensary for Diseases of the Ear, the institution became the first specialised institution strictly for aural diseases in Great Britain. It was framed as a social necessity, an alternative to the educational institutions for the deaf that had long denied the benefits of aural surgery. Moreover, the RDDE combated the general neglect by medical practitioners in treating disorders of the ear. This 'popular prejudice', Curtis argued, constructed deafness as an incurable affliction, a perspective that left deaf persons vulnerable to the claims of charlatans peddling miraculous wares. It also meant that, without access to proper inspection by a qualified aurist, children at institutions such as the London Asylum for the Deaf and Dumb (est. 1792) (LADD) were denied treatment for temporary hearing loss.

London society agreed with Curtis on the necessity of the RDDE and about the general neglect by medical practitioners. The *New Monthly Magazine* expressed the view that '[t]he pathology of the ear, neglected till of late, has now attained a vast importance by the institution', and congratulated Curtis for introducing the possibility that deafness could be cured.[16] Soho's clerks, domestic servants, needlewomen, artisans, distressed foreigners, soldiers, sailors, policemen, children and the deserving poor all sought advice and relief from the 'Prince of Ear Diseases' as the *Family Oracle of Health* ennobled Curtis.[17] The 'increasing utility' of the RDDE, another writer added, 'is daily manifested by a general success in the treatment of Deafness and other Diseases of the Ear not previously known in this country'.[18] In 1816, the RDDE's first year, 364 patients were admitted, 89 of whom were 'cured' and 75 'relieved' of their maladies. By the end of 1820, the dispensary had admitted 1,863 patients. With increased patronage and a growing list of subscriptions and patients, Curtis found larger premises at 10 Dean Street, Soho Square.[19]

From the start, Curtis appointed himself as Director and Aural Surgeon, with other practitioners joining as consultants. John Sims (1749–1831) was appointed as the first consulting physician, a position that would later be filled in the 1820s by Sir Henry Halford (1766–1844) and Sir Matthew John Tierney (1776–1845). The Prince Regent, crowned King George IV in 1820, remained the institution's foremost patron, although the Duke of Cumberland also extended support. As Nicholas Jewson has argued, by coaxing aristocratic patrons for favours, medical practitioners spurred fashionable trends in medicine to shape their careers and identities through their interactions with the laity rather than through their colleagues. This 'consultative relationship', as Jewson outlines, thus allowed the wealthy sick to exercise control over innovative treatments in their demands for a cure.[20] The governance guided by patrons could also frame the direction of the institution; however, subscriptions were required to manage daily expenses. Curtis personally solicited funds from prominent wealthy citizens, frequently through networks with which he connected via the circles of his socialite wife, Sophia Maria Newman, and from his own time in the Royal Navy.[21] Fund-raising literature was also distributed to solicit donations from charities and to project images of the RDDE as a humanitarian institution.[22]

According to Curtis, the RDDE was intended to serve two objectives. The primary objective was to provide charitable care, the 'relief of the industrious poor from a class of disease to the last degree painful and inconvenient, and often neglected, if not generally misunderstood'.[23] For patients whose hearing loss was too severe – cases diagnosed as 'irremediable' – hearing trumpets were supplied at a cost of seven shillings or free of charge. This provision is significant. On the one hand, it seemed to undermine the institution's ultimate goal of curing *all* cases of deafness; but, on the other hand, by supplying aids to make use of serviceable hearing, patients were still gaining acoustic function. Moreover, aids to hearing during this period were largely confined to the gentry and aristocracy, who were able to afford such extravagant devices.[24] The RDDE's distribution of aids to the poor provides an early instance of free provision that would later be embedded in the creation of the National Health Service and delivery of the Medresco Hearing Aid in post-war Britain.[25]

The second objective was to 'show that diseases of the ear, like diseases of other organs, if properly studied and judiciously treated, are by no means of so incurable or unmanageable a nature as it has been too much the custom to suppose'.[26] By presenting the RDDE as an institution for the clinical study of aural diseases as well as a place for experimentation in advanced treatment, Curtis hoped to attract talented scientific minds who would work on improving knowledge of the anatomy and physiology of the ear – with the hope that eventually deafness could be a completely obliterated disease.[27] Despite Curtis's second objective, however, out-patient care made up the bulk of treatment, and there is little evidence that any experimentation or clinical study took place at the RDDE prior to the 1870s. Several beds were installed in the 1830s for in-patient care, 'in order to accommodate ... not only infant deaf and dumb patients, but also persons from the country, and others ... who are destitute of a habitation in the metropolis'.[28]

As was standard with other medical institutions, patient admittance relied upon recommendation from either a consulting physician, a medical officer at the RDDE or a member of the Board of Governors. This practice continued until the 1870s, as did the Governors' right to nominate a candidate of their choice to be admitted for treatment free of charge.[29] Of particular interest to the Governors – and to Curtis – were infant or young patients. Medical practitioners were aware that deafness could be symptomatic, or a consequence, of certain kinds of childhood illnesses, including smallpox, measles and typhoid fever. On this note, Curtis claimed that if children were inspected for hearing loss as early as infancy, they had the greatest chance of receiving full restoration of hearing: the earlier a disease was diagnosed, the more likely deafness could be treated, if not prevented completely. Although few aurists agreed with Curtis's assertions at the time – William Wright (1773–1860) being a notable exception – by the end of the century James Kerr Love (1858–1942) had adopted this approach under the slogan 'prevention of deafness', urging school boards and public health organisations to implement systematic hearing tests for children. As a result of a study of children at the Glasgow Institute for the Deaf, Love reported that only 10 per cent of pupils were totally deaf. The majority had residual hearing, which, Love argued, could be utilised with the application of medical care or aids.[30]

The medical staff at the RDDE acted as agents of care, but their hearing-impaired patients were not always passive recipients or dependent objects of charity. Indeed, the RDDE records indicate that many patients actually sought care out of frustration or desperation over hearing loss, at times pleading to the Governors for a nomination for admission.[31] However, treatments of patients were not standardised; aurists made assessments based on inspection of the ears and an overview of patient history, but seemingly were also guided by patient responses, particularly in difficult cases. Seeking to standardise patient assessment, Curtis collaborated with his friend Dr Heinrich Schmaltz of Dresden to formulate a series of questions for obtaining a full and detailed patient history.[32] However, such questions could be intimidating for patients, especially if their hearing loss was too severe for them to properly understand what was asked of them, or if they were too embarrassed by their condition.

An anecdote by Reverend J. Richardson about his 'deaf and nervous friend', for instance, suggests how the 'great aurist' could extend his authority to guide (intimidate) patients' responses. As Richardson recalled, his friend was too timid to oppose or contradict anyone, so would reply 'yes' or 'no' to everything, answering questions as he 'conjectured the answer to be desired'.[33] Hearing about Curtis's successful cases at the RDDE, Richardson encouraged his friend to apply for a consultation, even though he personally found that Curtis 'took patients by storm rather than by protracted advances'. The friend described his consultation:

> [Curtis] seated the patient in a chair in which patients were placed during examination, and after various questions proceeded thus:
> 'You hear what I say to-day better than you did yesterday?'
> 'Yes, sir.'
> 'You hear what I say without difficulty; don't you?'
> 'Yes, sir.'
> 'What's your name?'
> 'Yes, sir.'
> 'How old are you?'
> 'Yes, sir.'
> The practitioner was growing irate, the patient was trembling with fear, he could hear nothing, but concluded that his safety depended on the acquiescence of his responses. The practitioner was resolved not to be so easily satisfied; he pulled out his watch, and held it to the ear of the patient.
> 'Do you hear that watch tick?'
> 'Yes, sir.'
> 'That's a d____d lie, for it doesn't go.'
> The patient, though he could not hear the words of Mr. Curtis, was aware something was wrong. He got out of the chair and out of the house as fast as he could, and never troubled the owner of them again with his presence.[34]

Although Curtis spent most of his career arguing that it was the aurists' responsibility to counteract 'popular prejudice' by forging their skills as diagnosticians in order to solidify their surgical authority, this encounter begs the question whether a diagnostic assessment was forcibly imposed upon a patient. Diagnostic efficacy for determining whether a case of deafness was curable was difficult since the instruments used for assessments were often inadequate. Variations of aural specula, light illuminators and convex lens heavily depended on natural light and were nearly useless on cloudy days; furthermore, instruments aided by candlelight could distort images and lead to misdiagnosis.[35] Added to the fact that the structure of the ear is too intricate and complex to provide sufficient light for examination, it is probable Curtis's interrogation-style questions were used to enhance diagnostic objectivity for proficiency in diagnosis and thus improve patient care.

Curtis's *Cases Illustrative of the Treatment of Diseases of the Ear* (1822) provides some insight into the types of care patients received at the RDDE.[36] Out of fifty-eight cases he treated in 1821, thirteen were cases of childhood deaf and dumbness; eleven were nervous afflictions; eight were 'violent' noises in the head (tinnitus); and four were cases of polypus requiring surgical removal. The remaining cases included: inflammations, herpetic eruptions, ulcers, puriform discharges, blockages from cold or flu, insects or hardened cerumen (ear wax) lodged in the ear canal, enlarged tonsils or structural obstructions in the Eustachian tubes. There were also cases of deafness caused by accident or abuse, including damage by another physician's crude attempt at treatment and the results of loud explosions from warfare. Curtis's 'plan' for restoring hearing usually followed a regimen of blistering behind the ear combined with 'complete' syringing and a series of pharmaceuticals assigned over several weeks – typical medical care of the period, although Curtis generally avoided more invasive surgical remedies advocated by other aurists, such as Eustachian tube catheterisation.

Some of the patients' descriptions are noteworthy, providing insight into the variability of causes of hearing loss and recommended courses of treatment during the nineteenth century. They included the 'grotesque appearance' of George Robinson who, suffering from otitis (inflammation of the eardrum), frightened patients in the waiting room. Mr V. of Switzerland was sent to the Leamington spa near Warwick after a three-week course of treatment. Captain D suffered polypus in his left ear, but refused an invasive surgical operation to remove it, so Curtis had to resort to ligature. Mrs N was galvanised daily over the course of six months to treat her nervous deafness before arriving at the RDDE for consultation; it is unclear what new treatment she was prescribed, although the galvanic treatment was discontinued. Master P became deaf following a blow from a ruler inflicted by an usher at his school. Thomas Nevenson, a carpenter who fell from a scaffold, was treated with leeches to stop blood flowing from his ears. Five-year-old Miss P was so traumatised by a servant leaving her in a cellar that she was left deaf and dumb; Curtis diagnosed her condition as nervous deafness.

Perhaps most notably, the cases of two twenty-eight-year old men, Charles Vernon and James Butler, who were both former pupils at the LADD, supported the RDDE's medical agenda and Curtis's stance on the limitations of educational institutions for 'helping' the deaf. After all, not only were Vernon and Butler's deafness badly managed by the asylum's physician, but if they had been properly treated at a young age by a trained aurist they would have avoided the frustration

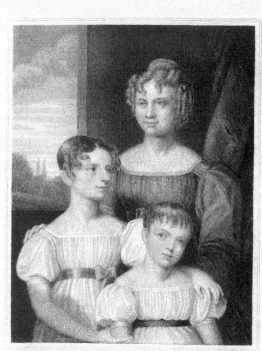

4.1 Selina Hewitt, Mary Ann Hauge and Mary Haines, allegedly 'successfully cured' at the Royal Dispensary for Diseases of the Ear. From: John Harrison Curtis, *An Essay on the Deaf and Dumb*, 2nd edn (London: Longman, 1834). Reproduced by permission of Yale University, Harvey Cushing/John Hay Whitney Medical Library.

of seeking a cure. As Curtis repeatedly stressed, it was more difficult to cure cases of deafness in adults than in children or infants.[37]

By 1823 a total of 3,500 patients have been received at the RDDE.[38] The increasing number of patients discharged as 'cured' or 'relieved' provided powerful ammunition for Curtis to undermine the validity of the popular prejudice. For, if deafness was curable, then there were no grounds for institutions like the LADD, or for sceptical medical practitioners to deny the authority of the specialised aurist. Although, like many medical practitioners, Curtis asserted his authority with his claims to cure, yet the concept of 'cure' itself is vexed when applied to deafness. As Catherine Kudlick argues, 'cure was something more likely to be bestowed than earned, something that came from outside rather than from within'.[39] For people with temporary loss of hearing brought about by a cold or blockages in the auditory canals, the relief can also only be temporary: when the cold returns, the deafness is no longer 'cured'. Likewise, for individuals who used ear trumpets or other kinds of acoustic aids, the 'cure' is effective only when the aid is in use.[40] When their aid is put away or not in use, the 'cured' patient is deaf once again.

Expansion and relocation: 1836–75

Despite the initial success of the RDDE and its overwhelming support from subscribers, by the mid-1830s the institution faced serious financial trouble. Curtis requested his more affluent patients to increase their subscriptions, while the Governors used the charitable imperative of the institution to solicit funds by offering incentives for patients.[41] For instance, on 25 February 1836 the Governors passed a resolution stating that any police constable afflicted with deafness could be admitted gratuitously for treatment. In addition, they sent out a statement declaring that soldiers and sailors could be admitted free of expense without requiring a letter of recommendation.[42]

Spoken and published church sermons were other recourses for persuading people to be charitable and contribute to the financial well-being of the RDDE. By outlining the RDDE's humanitarian pursuit in eradicating deafness, sermons attempted to convince parishioners of the institution's national and social value. They also provided the poor deaf with a platform to 'speak in voices louder than their own', although in so doing, they contributed to paternalist views of deafness.[43] As with many charitable imperatives for sensory disabilities, the deaf were perceived as vulnerable citizens at the mercy of hearing benefactors to rescue them from their exile, and religious discourses were 'highly influential in articulating otherness' to make disability a marked category, as Esme Cleall has argued.[44]

For instance, the Right Reverend Richard Ponsonby (1772–1853), bishop of Killaloe and Derry, delivered a sermon at St Martin-in-the-Field's church, preaching to aid the RDDE. His sermon was circulated with an introductory letter written by RDDE secretary Henry Sheppard Smyth, declaring a persistent need to 'awaken the sympathies of meek-eyed Charity' and raise awareness of the 'condition' of the deaf.[45] Ponsonby urged his congregation to support their 'dependent fellow-creatures', who 'have no voice to speak their misery' but who could be aided through the imperatives of the RDDE.[46] To stress this claim, he outlined how the RDDE exemplified the vast improvements made in aural surgery and how the progress made by its aurists actually improved the position of the deaf in society.

Charitable donations and philanthropic events such as *grandes fêtes champêtres*, organised to raise funds from the social elite, reveal the interwoven relationships between medical institutions, practitioners and Governors that relied heavily upon what Keir Waddington loosely terms 'benevolent economy'.[47] Since hospitals depended upon the voluntary ethic of their contributors, any financial crisis which the institution suffered 'was not simply a symptom of managerial inefficiency or failure to attract philanthropy' but, rather, a reflection on the availability of charitable resources.[48] Financial pressures from limited donations occasionally meant that Curtis and the RDDE's administrators had to extend their fund-raising campaigns towards other avenues: highlighting the institution's fashionable tastes, advertising the efficacy of treatments or promoting the reputation of its founder in order to encourage prominent society members to lend their social cachet.[49] Within medicine's gentlemanly circle, patronage by the social elite could be seen to confirm a practitioner's social standing and thus inspire increased donations, as it did in Curtis's case; however, it also meant that as long as Curtis's reputation was secured, so too was that of his institution.

In addition to the RDDE's fund-raising issues, two significant events occurred in the late 1830s that threatened its permanence. The first was the public disagreement between Curtis and the aural anatomist Joseph Toynbee (1815–69) over Curtis's use of creosote (pitch oil) as a treatment for deafness caused by lack of wax formation. This 'deficiency of the secretion' of wax, according to Curtis, was the most common cause of deafness, a statement which Toynbee furiously disagreed with, accusing Curtis of gross incompetency, fraud and duping the public on the potential curability of deafness.[50] To distance themselves from any potential fall-outs from the scandal, the Governors requested Curtis to remove himself as Director, although they honoured his contributions and Curtis was allowed to advertise himself as 'Surgeon to the Dispensary'.[51] Such diatribes indicate that Curtis was an important public figure – the very face of the RDDE – and was expected to behave with a certain decree of decorum and respectability. The Governors clearly feared Curtis's deteriorating reputation and were concerned that the frequent accusations of quackery made against him would harm the goodwill of the institution. This dismissal and a series of bankruptcies eventually led Curtis to sell the RDDE in 1841 to the aurist William Harvey (1806–76), who was then tasked by the Governors to 'talk away the ugly face of the Royal Dispensary'.[52]

The second event was the death of King George IV in 1830 and then of King William IV in 1837, both long-time patrons of the RDDE, whose absences threatened the future stability of the institution. In 1838, on behalf of the Governors, Smyth petitioned the newly crowned Queen Victoria to acknowledge official patronage and continue royal support. Smyth's letter stressed that valuable social service would perish if the RDDE lost the necessary funds to sustain itself: the 'grounds on which we solicit this favour are in its extensive usefulness to the poor classes', as well as its service to civic employees.[53] Coupled with a petition signed by the Governors, Smyth explained that the 'best evidence of extensive good which the poor have derived from the Dispensary, consists in the fact, that since its institution upwards of ten thousand two hundred and forty patients have been admitted to its advantages, very many of whom have by its instrumentality been relieved from maladies which had incapacitated them from following their occupation.'[54] A letter from Smyth to the Earl of Harewood reveals that the petition was not granted immediately. Smyth thus requested Harewood to use his influence with Sir Robert Peel (1788–1850) and other persons close to the Queen to urge acceptance of another petition on behalf of the RDDE.[55] On 5 December 1842, at the request of the Duke of Cambridge, Queen Victoria became the official patroness of the RDDE.

As patronage secured the RDDE's future, the transforming state of aural surgery and the professionalisation of aurists shifted approaches to the diagnosis and treatment of hearing disorders. However, discussions about cases were not strictly confined to medical diagnosis; alongside descriptions of deafness caused by herpes, accidents, smallpox or syphilis, aurists theorised that deafness could be the result of immoral lifestyles, poor dietary choices or unsanitary living conditions.[56] They also debated demarcations between congenital and acquired deafness, recognising that serious cases of deaf-mutism were formidable and that successful treatments depended on individualised case studies. This was not necessarily a new perspective but, rather, a strengthening of professional boundaries during the 1840s and 1850s guided by aurists' quest to define the parameters of their speciality and distance themselves from 'quack-aurists'. Toynbee, for instance, argued that it was necessary to reform 'the very degraded state of aural surgery; the practice of which had, through its neglect by legitimate practitioners, become synonymous with charlatans'.[57]

Under the directorship of William Harvey, the RDDE embraced the new empirical framework for pathological studies, particularly for understanding deaf-mutism. Aurists were becoming increasingly aware that medical treatment was limited, if not completely ineffective, for deaf-mutes, but hoped that anatomical research could reveal causes of the affliction and provide new avenues for surgically treating hearing disorders. James Yearsley (1805–66), for instance, focused his research on the relationship between the throat and the ear, claiming that the relationship between the two organs could provide valuable information about the acoustic mechanism of the ear. His work on tonsils was particularly influential to physicians at the RDDE; records dating to the early 1830s show that tonsils and adenoid operations, as devised by Yearsley, were routine procedures.

The increase of anatomical dissections and compilation of statistics also provided aurists with new frameworks or thinking about how to medically or surgically cultivate hearing power. Toynbee published a report outlining 1,532 dissections of the ear, with specimens obtained from the LADD, from the Asylum for Idiots at Earlswood, Surrey and from donations and collections from patients.[58] His work asserted that if no evidence of residual hearing was found in examination or after treatment – especially in children – then alternative recourses were to be recommended: being educated as deaf-mutes or given ear trumpets to excite the 'nervous stimulation' of the ears. By the 1850s both practices were implemented at the RDDE. While it is difficult to assess the number of patients proved to be 'incurable' – annual reports certainly favoured more successful cases – at least two-fifths of patients admitted to the RDDE were marked as 'curable', even those whose cases were of the 'most hopeless character and of protracted duration'.[59] Like Curtis, Harvey explained that the prognosis of deafness and diseases of the ear relied on diagnosis at an early age in order to be subjected to judicious and favourable treatment. It was imperative for patients to seek out an aurist as soon as symptoms of hearing loss were present, or else disease is 'allowed to run its course unchecked, or is rendered incurable by mismanagement'.[60]

Here, it is implied that deafness was the patient's responsibility: if the ailment was incurable, it was not because the aurist's skills were limited but because the patient waited too long to seek out proper treatment or sought treatment from an unqualified practitioner who, unfortunately, made the ailment worse. Despite the profession's shift in accepting that some cases were 'incurable', the contradictory approach towards treatment reveals how aurists were still adamant in claiming that deafness was a disease that could be eliminated. For instance, while many of Harvey's cases at the RDDE were individuals with 'temporary deafness' – whom we now call 'hard of hearing' – he refers to deaf-mutism as an 'evil' that necessitated urgent and demanding treatment by any means necessary. He accepted some cases as 'incurable', but at the same time he argued that statistics should be utilised by the aurist to identify various causes of deaf-mutism to determine whether a cure was possible. After all, about 14,000 deaf and dumb persons were living in England, and, presumably, many went without proper treatment.[61]

Transformation as a surgical centre: 1876–1900

In 1878, as the lease for the building on Dean Street was about to expire, the Governors of the RDDE decided to move to new premises on 66 Firth Street. An increase in patients and a growing waiting list rendered the former location inadequate to serve the purposes of the institution.[62] When the RDDE relocated, it was also renamed to reflect its status as a specialised surgical centre for aural diseases; henceforth it was known as the Royal Ear Hospital. Urban Pritchard (1845–1926), who was appointed as Assistant Surgeon in 1874, became Director after Harvey's death in 1876; he was also elected to Senior Surgeon and held the post until 1900, overseeing the surgical team at the hospital. Farquhar Matheson (1840–1905) was Assistant Surgeon and, in 1880, became Surgeon to the Hospital. While Harvey had spent much of his role at the RDDE ensuring finances were stabilised and reconstructing its reputation as a skilled, qualified and beneficial institution for the treatment of aural diseases, Pritchard aimed to advance the hospital into a new surgical age that promised innovative treat-ments for patients.

Pritchard's agenda was to provide aural surgery with a strong institutional base to exert its authority over hearing loss, an influence that he also extended to his other appointments. At King's College London he was appointed dem-onstrator of practical anatomy in 1872; fourteen years later, he was appointed Professor of Aural Surgery, the only chair of its kind in England. Hospital and university positions not only represented status but promoted professionalisation, which Pritchard used to place British aural surgery in a strong position on the international stage.[63] From 1884 to 1922 he served as the British representative of the organising committee of the International Congress of Otology; in 1899 he was elected President of the British Otological Society, and from 1901 to 1903 was second president of the Otological Section of the Royal Society of Medicine. Pritchard also served as editor of *International Archives of Otology*, using the journal as a platform for discussing new advancements in aural surgery and the classification of ear diseases, including his research with Arthur H. Cheatle (1867–1929) into the histology of the labyrinth and anatomy of the temporal bone.

Records of the hospital during the closing years of the nineteenth century are limited, but there is strong evidence that Pritchard not only devoted himself to clinical work and his private practice, but also influenced important administrative changes at the hospital.[64] By 1880 the hospital had reconfigured the role of the surgeon, limiting his role in managing daily affairs. The Governors decided that the hospital should be conducted as an entirely public institution, with the Senior Surgeon's control restricted to the surgical staff only, rather than being over the entire hospital as had been the case for Curtis and Harvey. The honoraria that surgeons received were also fixed so that they no longer received fees directly from patients, but from the superintendent of the hospital, who was responsible for managing the finances of the institution. These changes were presented as necessary to ensure the financial stability of the hospital, which up to that point had relied heavily on the donations of subscribers.[65]

Other changes were directed towards the well-being of patients. Previously, the institution had functioned mainly as an out-patient centre, with reserved beds for serious surgical cases requiring hospitalisation. A new in-patient department was built with separate wards for men, women and children; private wards were also available for affluent patients. The out-patient department was refitted for tonsil and adenoid operations. Additional positions were created to expand the staff, including the appointments of Edward Cresswell Baber (1850–1919) and Arthur Cheatle as assistant surgeons to Pritchard in 1893. While these changes greatly advanced the usefulness of the institution and its commitment to providing safe surgical care and treatment, they also considerably increased the annual expenditure of the hospital, straining available charity funds; legacies from patients as well as fees were crucial in ensuring the livelihood of the hospital and its staff.

By 1890, upwards of 138,000 patients had been admitted to the hospital since its founding in 1816. To surgeons at the hospital, the number of patients being cured or relieved was proof of the progress of medical incursions into deafness. The more access aural surgeons had to deaf bodies and a variety of deafness cases, the better they were able to diagnose the type of hearing impairment and to dispense treatment. It was imperative, the surgeons argued, that young children were examined as early as possible – statistical records revealed that one of every hundred children of school age required treatment at the Royal Ear Hospital. As Jan Branson and Don Miller have argued, the medical approach to the 'problem of deafness' during the Victorian period placed deafness into a site of pathology. Diagnostic procedures particularly contributed to the developments of normality, disability and pathology, concepts that drastically influenced Deaf resistance to oralism and its stance on normalising deaf persons through speech.[66] To aurists, however, oralism represented a scientific advancement, an approach for validating their authority over deaf bodies.

As aural surgeons obtained more insight into the anatomy and pathology of the ear, they became aware of the stark distinctions between deafened persons and deaf-mutes. Some recognised that medical incursions into deaf-mutes were unhelpful, but others, like Harvey and Pritchard, argued that educators could make up for the limitations of medicine after all medical avenues were exhausted. Technological assistance was also recommended for those with minimal hearing power, but there is little evidence that the hospital continued to supply ear trumpets after its relocation to Firth Street; indeed, not until the 1930s did the hospital recreate the same free provision of aids for patients as had been established by Curtis. Pritchard and Cheatle did prescribe different kinds of acoustic aids for their patients, including the artificial eardrum for patients with tympanic perforation. However, they made it clear that technological assistance was not a complete replacement for proper medical treatment: medicine was still advancing, so these aids could be mere temporary measures for deaf persons to interact with hearing society.

Conclusions

By drawing national attention to the importance of medically treating deafness, the RDDE played a significant role in increasing the authority of aurists and affirming their jurisdiction over the deaf population.[67] Medical treatment of patients demonstrated not only that the majority of cases of hearing impairment were curable but that the claims of those who propelled the 'popular prejudice' argument were tenuous. The institution's founder, John Harrison Curtis, intended to provide a base for aural surgery to develop, expand and address new techniques for treating deafness, while also providing opportunities for clinical study of the ears. His mandate was carried forward and expanded by William Harvey and Urban Pritchard, both of whom also promoted the RDDE as offering a medical infrastructure for ensuring that deafness was appropriately managed and treated.

The history of the RDDE thus provides insight for studying how medical practitioners sought to extend their authority and medicalise deafness by aligning with the oralist campaign. Although the archival collections of the institution are limited, it is possible to view this connection through other aural hospitals in London, particularly the Institution for Diseases of the Ear founded by James Yearsley in 1838, which later became the Metropolitan Ear, Nose and Throat Hospital. However, by adding a disability perspective, as Catherine Kudlick urges, the notion of cure as advocated by aurists becomes reconstructed as a 'shorthand for an idea that few recognise as a fragile promise'; most deaf people could never completely recover their hearing – and for those born deaf, they could never fully hear sounds, if at all.[68]

What the oralist focus on speech as advocated by aurists tells us, moreover, is how medical specialists created opportunities for themselves to participate in conversations about deaf education at the turn of the century and to advocate the prospect of 'normalising' deaf people by supporting medical advances in hearing tests and devices for amplifying hearing power. In so doing, the RDDE was promoted as a 'world-focusing point for the most advanced knowledge' of aural diseases, for aural surgery was 'on the threshold of a new era. Deafness can be termed the "Cinderella of diseases," for few realise the disability it imposes. The number of the deaf is on the increase, especially in juvenile cases, and there is great national work to be done.'[69]

Notes

1 Royal Ear Hospital Archives, The National Archives, Kew (henceforth REH Archives), UCH/MED/H/REH/11, Pamphlet, University College Hospital Collections, *He that Hath Ears To Hear*.

2 J. H. Curtis, *A Clinical Report of the Royal Dispensary for Diseases of the Ear* (London: Longman, Rees, Orme, Browne, Green, &c., 1832), p. 4.

3 R. A. R. Edwards, *Words Made Flesh: Nineteenth-century Deaf Education and the Growth of Deaf Culture* (New York, NY and London: New York University Press, 2012); D. C. Baynton, *Defectives in the Land: Disability and Immigration in the Age of Eugenics* (Chicago, IL: University of Chicago Press, 2016).

4 J. Esmail, *Reading Victorian Deafness: Signs and Sounds in Victorian Literature and Culture* (Athens, OH: Ohio University Press, 2013).

5 C. Kudlick, 'Social history of medicine and disability history', in M. Rembis, C. Kudlick and K. E. Nielsen (eds), *The Oxford Handbook of Disability History* (Oxford: Oxford University Press, 2018), pp. 105–24.

6 J. A. Brune and D. J. Wilson, *Disability and Passing: Blurring the Lines of Identity* (Philadelphia, PA: Temple University Press, 2012).

7 For a sociological and historical overview of deafness and medicalisation, see: L. Mauldin, *Made to Hear: Cochlear Implants and Raising Deaf Children* (Minneapolis, MN: University of Minnesota Press, 2016), pp. 5–15.

8 On social images, see: A. T. Quartararo, *Deaf Identity and Social Images in Nineteenth-century France* (Washington, DC: Gallaudet University Press, 2008).

9 J. P. Anderson, *War, Disability and Rehabilitation in Britain* (Manchester: Manchester University Press, 2011); B. Linker, 'On the borderland of medical and disability history: a survey of the fields', *Bulletin of the History of Medicine*, 87:4 (2013), 499–535.

10 C. McGuire, 'The 'Deaf Subscriber' and the Shaping of the British Post Office's Amplified Telephones 1919–1939' (PhD thesis, University of Leeds, 2016).

11 C. Rosenberg, 'Social class and medical care in nineteenth-century America', *Journal of the History of Medicine*, 29:1 (1974), 32–54; S. Cherry, *Medical Services and the Hospital in Britain, 1860–1939* (Cambridge: Cambridge University Press, 1996); B. Croxson, 'The public and private faces of eighteenth-century London dispensary charity', *Medical History*, 41 (1997), 127–49; G. B. Carruthers and L. A. Carruthers, *A History of Britain's Hospitals* (Leicester: The Book Guild, 2005); M. Higgs, *Life in the Victorian Hospital* (Stroud: The History Press, 2009).

12 L. Granshaw, '"Fame and fortune by means of bricks and mortar": the medical profession and specialist hospitals in Britain, 1800–1948', in L. Granshaw and R. Porter (eds), *The Hospital in History* (London and New York, NY: Routledge, 1989), pp. 199–220; L. Granshaw, 'The rise of the modern hospital in Britain', in A. Wear (ed.), *Medicine in Society: Historical Essays* (Cambridge: Cambridge University Press, 1992).

13 Esmail, *Reading Victorian Deafness*, p. 166.

14 On John Harrison Curtis's stint in the Royal Navy, see: Jaipreet Virdi [as Virdi-Dhesi], '"From the Hands of Quacks": Deafness, Aural Surgery and the Making of a Surgical Speciality in 19th Century London' (PhD thesis, University of Toronto, 2014).

15 'John Harrison Curtis', in Anonymous, *Authentic Memoirs, Biographical, Critical and Literary of the most eminent physicians and surgeons in Great Britain*, 2nd edn (London: Sherwood, Neely & Jones, 1818), p. 536.

16 *The New Monthly Magazine*, 8 (1 October 1817), p. 237.

17 Anonymous, '35th Annual Meeting of the Dispensary', *The London Lancet*, 2 (1852), 154; *The Family Oracle of Health: Economy, Medicine, and Good Living*, 8 (1824), p. 329.

18 A. Highmore, *Philanthropia metropolitana: a view of the charitable institutions established in and near London, chiefly during the last twelve years* (London: Longman, Hurst, Rees, Orme, and Brown, 1822), p. 355.

19 Curtis, *A Clinical Report*, p. 8.

20 N. D. Jewson, 'Medical knowledge and the patronage system in 18th century England', *Sociology*, 8 (1974), 369–85.

21 Family Search, 'England marriages 1538–1973', www.Familysearch.org.

22 Croxson, 'The public and private faces', 130.

23 J. H. Curtis, *A Clinical Report of the Royal Dispensary for Diseases of the Ear* (London: T. and G. Underwood, 1827).

24 G. Gooday and K. Sayer, *Managing the Experience of Hearing Loss in Britain, 1830–1930* (London: Palgrave Macmillan, 2017).

25 Medresco (contraction of 'Medical Research Council') was the first hearing aid developed in conjunction with the Medical Research Council, the National Health Service and the National Institute for the Deaf in the 1930s and 1940s. For an overview of its history, see: McGuire, 'The "Deaf Subscriber"' and S. McNally, 'Medresco: The History of State Sponsored Auditory Assistance' (PhD thesis, University of Leeds PhD, forthcoming).

26 Curtis, *A Clinical Report*, p. 12.

27 J. H. Curtis, *An Introductory Lecture, as delivered 1816 at the Royal Dispensary for Disease of the Ear* (London: W. Clowes, 1818).

28 Curtis, *A Clinical Report*, p. 3.

29 Highmore, *Philanthropia metropolitana*, p. 355.

30 J. K. Love, *Deaf-Mutism: A Clinical and Pathological Study* (Glasgow: J. MacLehose and Sons, 1896).

31 REH Archives, UCH/MED/H/REH, Committee Papers.

32 J. H. Curtis, *Advice to the Deaf: The Present State of Aural Surgery*, 5th edn (London: Whitaker and Co., 1845).

33 J. Richardson, *Recollections, Political, Literary, Dramatic, and Miscellaneous of the Last half-Century*, Volume II (London: C. Mitchell, 1856), p. 290.

34 *Ibid.*, pp. 291–2.

35 J. Virdi [as Virdi-Dhesi], 'Curtis's Cephaloscope: deafness and the making of surgical authority in London, 1815–1845', *Bulletin of the History of Medicine*, 87:3 (2013), 364–5.

36 J. H. Curtis, *Cases Illustrative of the Treatment of Diseases of the Ear, both local and constitutional* (London: T. and G. Underwood, 1822).

37 *Ibid.*

38 Anonymous, *The Annual Subscription Charities and Public Societies in London* (London: John Murray, 1823), p. 31.

39 Kudlick, 'Social history of medicine and disability history', p. 114.

40 On the concept of 'cures' and of the curative, see: B. J. Venkat, 'Cures', *Public Culture*, 28:3 (2016), 475–97.

41 REH Archives, UCH/MED/H/REH/4/5, Letter to J.H. Curtis, 20 February 1837.

42 British Library (hereafter BL), Ms 40499, f.129, Letter from Colonel Rowan to Henry Sheppard Smyth, 1838; BL, Ms 40499, f.193, Petition to Queen Victoria from the Governors of the Royal Dispensary for Diseases of the Ear, 1838.

43 D. Andrew, 'Two medical charities in eighteenth-century London: the Lock Hospital and the Lying-in Charity for Married Women', in J. Barry and C. Jones (eds), *Medicine and Charity before the Welfare State* (London and New York, NY: Routledge, 1991), pp. 82–97, at p. 83.

44 E. Cleall, '"Deaf to the word": gender, deafness and Protestantism in nineteenth-century Britain and Ireland', *Gender & History*, 25:5 (2013), 590–603, at 591.

45 R. Ponsonby, *A Sermon Preached … in aid of the Royal Dispensary for Diseases of the Ear* (London: J. G. and F. Rivington, 1834).

46 *Ibid.*, p. 9.

47 K. Waddington, *Charity and the London Hospitals, 1850–1898* (London: Royal Historical Society, 2000).

48 *Ibid.*, p. 3.

49 F. K. Prochaska, 'Charity bazaars in nineteenth-century England', *The Journal of British Studies*, 16:2 (1977), 62–84.

50 For further details on this debate, see: Virdi, 'Curtis's Cephaloscope'; A. Mudry, 'The making of a career: Joseph Toynbee's first steps in otology', *Journal of Laryngology and Otology*, 126:1 (2012), 2–7.
51 Sources conflict on the exact nature of his exit; some say he resigned, while others claim he was forced into retirement. 'Royal Dispensary for Diseases of the Ear –Retirement of Mr Curtis', *Essex Standard* (1847).
52 J. F. Clarke, 'The career of a specialist: John Harrison Curtis, aurist', in *Autobiographical Recollections of the Medical Profession* (London: J. and A. Churchill, 1874), p. 370.
53 BL, Ms 404499, f.193, Petition to Queen Victoria.
54 *Ibid.*
55 BL, Ms 40499, f.191, Letter from Henry Shepard Smyth to Lord Harewood, n.d. [1841].
56 Esmail, *Reading Victorian Deafness*, pp. 166–7.
57 Anonymous, 'Westminster Medical Society. Saturday, October 26th, 1839: Dr. Chowne, President', *The Lancet*, 33:845 (1839), 239.
58 J. Toynbee, *The Deaf and Dumb: Their Condition, Education, and Medical Treatment* (London: John Churchill, 1858).
59 W. Harvey, *The Ear in Health and Disease* (London: Henry Renshaw, 1854), p. 39.
60 *Ibid.*
61 *Ibid.*
62 J. H. Cardwell, *Two Centuries of Soho* (London: Truslove and Hanson, 1898), pp. 70–1.
63 Waddington, *Charity and the London Hospitals*, p. 12; A. Digby, *Making a Medical Living: Doctors and Patients in the English Market for Medicine, 1720–1911* (Cambridge: Cambridge University Press, 2002); M. J. Peterson, *The Medical Profession in Mid-Victorian London* (Berkeley, CA: University of California Press, 1978).
64 REH Archives, UCH/MED/H/REH, Royal Ear Hospital Committee Papers.
65 REH Archives, UCH/MED/H/REH/3–4, Royal Ear Hospital Minutes of Governors Meeting and Annual Reports.
66 J. Branson and D. Miller, *Damned for Their Difference: The Cultural Construction of Deaf People as Disabled* (Washington, DC: Gallaudet University Press, 2002), p. 88.
67 On the concept of jurisdiction and medical authority, see: A. Abbott, *The System of the Profession: An Essay on the Division of Expert Labor* (Chicago, IL: University of Chicago Press, 1988).
68 Kudlick, 'Social history of medicine and disability history', p. 116.
69 REH, *He that Hath Ears To Hear.*

5

DRUNKENNESS, DEGENERATION AND DISABILITY IN ENGLAND

Joanne Woiak

Discourses and policies that connected the concepts of alcoholism and degeneration were prominent sites at which disability was constructed in the Victorian and Edwardian eras. Alcoholism was perceived as a 'borderland' disability, the boundaries of which were defined in distinct ways by members of various groups of professionals and reformers. Physicians, psychiatrists, temperance advocates and eugenicists promoted and contested a variety of ideas about the aetiology and effects of inebriety. These medical and eugenic discourses focused on two questions that linked alcohol to disability: how was susceptibility to heavy drinking connected to conditions that were labelled insanity and mental deficiency, and how could parental drunkenness produce offspring that were identified as constitutionally weak and feeble-minded?

The disease concept of inebriety was initially promoted in the 1880s, under the auspices of the Society for the Study of Inebriety (SSI), to explain alcoholism as a type of mental illness and therefore a problem that fell within the domain of the psychiatric profession.[1] Around 1900, the linkage between the concepts of alcoholism and racial degeneration shifted to a focus on hereditary effects and maternity, so that excessive drinking was identified as both a cause and a symptom of disability, and the problem was to be dealt with by eugenicists, public health doctors and state policy makers.[2] In both eras, the borderland of alcoholism served to legitimise professional expertise and institutional control over populations implicated in the alcohol problem.

However, considerably different policies for institutionalisation and drink control were implemented in each era, resulting in disparate impacts on people's lives, depending on their social class and gender. In the late nineteenth century, private medical retreats were licensed for voluntary treatment of affluent, male inebriates.[3] The disease concept of inebriety served the interests of both psychiatrists and those families who sought relief from the social stigma associated with alcoholism. After the turn of the century, attention turned to the female figures termed the habitual drunkard and the working-class unfit mother. About 4,000 poor, alcoholic women were diagnosed as mentally defective and sentenced indefinitely within the inebriate reformatory system that operated from 1898 until 1913.[4] These institutions offered an alternative to criminal incarceration, but explicitly aimed to control these women's perceived moral deviancy through surveillance and removal. Many other women whose drinking was considered socially dangerous found themselves classified as not disabled and therefore not deserving of assistance. Their deficiencies as mothers and their children's disabilities were instead attributed to personal incompetence, while their situations of domestic and economic distress were relatively disregarded.

The history of alcoholism illustrates ways that disability was shaped as a category for medical and policy action in distinct socio-political contexts through the interplay between intersecting social identities, professional and administrative interests and public discourses about social problems. The associations drawn between disability and drinking were both determined by, and contributed to shaping, the identity systems and ideologies of gender and class in Victorian and Edwardian England. Alcoholism was defined as a borderland condition demarcated from, but closely adjacent to, the more firmly established disability classifications of insanity and mental deficiency. Within the landscapes of medicine and public policy, inebriety occupied an intermediate territory between pathology and vice, between biological and environmental causation and between curable and incurable condition. Those individuals labelled as problematic drunkards lived at the vigilantly patrolled boundary between deserving and undeserving recipients of medical care and social supports.

Borderlands of alcoholism: demarcation and control

Activists in the teetotal movement from the 1830s and the medical temperance movement from the 1860s linked alcoholism to disability through their research and propaganda on the physiological and mental harm caused by long-term heavy drinking.[5] By the 1870s, hereditarian psychiatrists theorised that alcohol was a 'brain poison' that caused insanity across generations, while a distinct group of medical experts proposed that inebriety should be recognised as a physical disease because it involved a hereditary predisposition to multiple forms of mental instability.[6] Recent historical writing has especially focused on how the medicalisation of alcoholism as a kind of mental disability, which lay outside the drinker's control, contested and complicated presuppositions about morality, responsibility and free will.[7]

With the acceptance of Social Darwinist and eugenic ideology at the turn of the century contributing to the 'crisis of national efficiency', eugenicists and public health professionals renewed the focus on heredity and provided evidence that parental drinking could directly injure offspring both before and after birth. They advocated for drink-control measures, reforming of maternal hygiene, education in 'race betterment' and compulsory institutionalisation. Existing scholarship in medical, social and policy history has addressed some of the ways in which expert and popular discourses connected the concept of alcoholism and the alcohol problem with anxieties about racial degeneration and national deterioration.[8] The history of legislative solutions for the treatment and control of alcoholism (the 1879 Habitual Drunkards Act and the 1898 Inebriates Act), along with questions about who ran the institutions under these policies and who was incarcerated, have also been explored in some depth for specific geographical regions.[9]

A critical disability studies lens can further elaborate the history of ideas and practices around inebriety, disability and treatment regimes. Disability studies demonstrates how social and professional preoccupations with alcohol use, represented in theories and policies propounded by different actors, coalesced in the making of mental disability in Victorian and Edwardian England. In contrast to historical approaches that treat mental deficiency as 'provid[ing] a symbol that linked overlapping anxieties about moral, demographic, and racial decline', disability history takes seriously both the lived experience of disabled people and the social construction of categories of disability.[10] Answering Beth Linker's call for bringing disability 'front and center to be fully theorised and systematically studied', the current project situates the history of alcoholism at the 'borderland' between the disciplines of disability history and medical history by infusing a disability studies perspective into a topic previously addressed mainly by medical and social historians.[11]

Mark Jackson's work on 'the borderland of imbecility' offers an especially useful analytical framework for developing a disability history of inebriety and intemperance. Jackson notes that the word 'borderland' was employed in the late-Victorian and Edwardian period to describe the sometimes blurry boundary between disease and health, as well as 'conditions or behaviour that lay between, and sometimes served to connect, disparate clinical and social pathologies'.[12] Specifically analysing the social uses of the concepts of imbecility and feeble-mindedness from 1890 to 1914, Jackson poses 'inter-related questions about the ways in which boundaries were established between "normal" and "pathological"' and considers how these labels 'served to link contemporary conceptions of mental deficiency, criminality, poverty and promiscuity'.[13] Feeble-mindedness and imbecility were constructed as 'borderline states of deficiency', distinguishable from normality on the one side and more 'severe' mental disability on the other, but representing a 'discrete, pathological but manageable menace to society'.[14] The presence of feeble-minded people was threatening because they were not yet identified and contained through institutionalisation.

A similar argument could be made about the identification and regulation of inebriety in its late-Victorian and Edwardian formulations: alcoholism was a troubling borderland condition because it was ambiguous, unruly and unconstrained. How 'abnormal' were that borderland's inhabitants in terms of the prevalence and severity of their condition, and therefore how threatening were they to themselves, their families, society, the nation or the human race? How should they be managed? Inebriety and imbecility were defined somewhat indeterminately as existing somewhere between the standards of normal and pathological. Yet both entities were also presumed to be chief causes of many social ills, and medical professionals sought to justify their role as experts in solving those problems through diagnosis, treatment and new institutional provisions.

Christine Crabbe's 2014 thesis, 'On the Borderland of Insanity: Women, Dipsomania and Inebriety, 1879–1913', deploys Jackson's concept to examine medical and legislative apparatuses that framed women habitual drunkards as 'in need of care or protection' because they were 'doubtful cases' who did not quite fit the diagnostic categories of insanity or idiocy.[15] Crabbe illustrates that inebriety was seen as lying in an 'ambiguous zone' up until 1913, when many habitual drunkards became classified as feeble-minded under the Mental Deficiency Act and most of the inebriate reformatories were therefore closed.[16] 'The concept of the borderland was useful for medical officers, proprietors and managers of inebriate reformatories because it provided a figurative space to assess and evaluate the inmates in their care ... as either hopeful or hopeless' in terms of treatment.[17] Crabbe's work focuses on discourses and practices that impacted on women who received services, offering an important perspective that, for some, or even many of these patients, the regimes within the reformatories may have provided necessary support, not just social control.[18]

Victorian psychiatrists such as Henry Maudsley (1835–1918), a prominent proponent of the hereditarian basis of mental disability, had used the language of 'a borderland between sanity and insanity' to posit an intermediary zone of ambiguously classified medical conditions that included 'epilepsy, neuralgia, chorea, and dipsomania'.[19] Alcoholism – then medically termed 'dipsomania' or 'inebriety' – was also sometimes described as having an intermediate status between insanity and crime. Psychiatrists and other physicians took a variety of stances that either corroborated or contested the meanings of alcoholism and problem drinking that had been promulgated by the temperance movement since the 1810s.[20] Since intemperance could be addressed using differing emphases on its physical, mental and moral causes and effects, the line between conceptualising it as disease or as vice (expressed as sin, character flaw or crime) was always fluid. As the title of Maudsley's monograph illustrated, alcoholism represented one borderland where there were conflicting medical theories and popular beliefs about patients' 'responsibility in mental disease' and about who was deserving of treatment and care.[21]

After the turn of the century, discourse on the drink problem became primarily entangled with escalating public health and eugenic concerns about infant mortality, maternal 'fecklessness' and differential birth rates of citizens deemed fit versus unfit. Cries of alarm were raised about the high rejection rate of Boer War recruits, which many commentators linked to the idea of hereditary deterioration of the population.[22] As in the prior era, Edwardian medical and legal discourses continued to grapple with whether the borderland of inebriety should be dealt with as disability or vice; accordingly, historians have interpreted the treatment practices offered in the inebriate reformatories as semi-penal.[23] However, Edwardian doctors and reformers were clear about their target population for 'reform': the 1898 Inebriates Act was significantly gendered, in that disproportionate numbers of women were sentenced and confined.

Popular rhetoric, scientific theories and state policies coalesced to define poor and working-class femininity as reproductive: women served the national welfare as producers of labourers and soldiers. Of course, working-class women, and men, were also supposed to be productively *working*. Political and medical systems were created to maintain the separation between the work-based and need-based distributive systems, 'defining and redefining the boundaries of dependency by establishing categories which expressed "a culturally legitimate rationale for nonparticipation in the labor system"'.[24]

As Deborah Stone's work has shown, states deploy disability as one of the key rationales for 'dependency'. Anne Borsay's historical overview of the British institutions that created and controlled disability does not include the systems of inebriate retreats and reformatories. But when the borderland medical diagnosis of inebriety morphed into an 'official category of disability' via those medical and social control apparatuses, the label 'inebriate' functioned as another mechanism to demarcate the 'deserving' welfare and treatment recipients from those who were deemed capable of productive contributions to society.[25] Receiving care in the early twentieth-century reformatories was fundamentally about subduing deviancy through incarceration of the poor, which paralleled the purposes of the need-based workhouse, mental hospital and idiot asylum. The borderland of alcoholism concomitantly served to exclude the 'undeserving' mass of lower-class women who were seen as not legitimately in need of financial assistance or care provisions, but who were nonetheless stigmatised as drunkards and unfit mothers.

Much like imbecility, the borderland of alcoholism represented a novel medical and administrative category for delineating and regulating dependency and deviancy, while also serving as a connecting category. Drunkenness was readily implicated as an underlying cause or co-occurring condition with other social ills, such as pauperism, prostitution, criminality and mental deficiency. In short, inebriety and imbecility were entities similarly 'situated at the borders of a bewildering variety of domains', which could therefore be deployed for many social, political and professional ends.[26]

The disease of inebriety: hereditary degeneration and personal responsibility

The 'drink problem' in England was first addressed by reformers committed to the principle of total abstinence, and later by the temperance movement. Many of the leaders of the anti-alcohol movement (1820–60) were working-class men, although a few voices were raised from the ranks of the medical profession. Anglo-American teetotal and medical temperance tracts and lectures written by prominent abstaining medical practitioners described drunkenness as both a social and a medical scourge, and expounded on the physiological and pathological effects of alcohol consumption. However, these works only briefly mentioned observations and beliefs about the problems associated with heredity, including debility in the offspring of drinkers, the heritability of the drink habit and how the temperance reformation might improve the well-being of future as well as current generations.[27]

Mid-nineteenth-century temperance reformers and doctors who were interested in the medical-scientific aspects of the alcohol problem focused on the control and treatment of male drinkers, or, as one historian of the American temperance movement put it, on 'manhood lost'.[28] Intemperate working-class husbands and fathers were said to be a destructive influence because of wasted wages and earning power. Leaders thus appealed to men's notions of 'respectability' and self-improvement in order to regulate both alcohol use and the meanings of masculinity.[29]

In the 1870s medical organisations, first in the United States, then in Britain, were formed for the study and cure of what they termed the 'physical disease of inebriety.[30] The small group of British experts who comprised the SSI maintained that alcohol abuse was a nervous disease that afflicted people 'of both sexes and all walks of life'. However, those individuals differed from the common drunkard in that they were 'branded with the red-hot iron of alcoholic heredity'.[31]

Norman Kerr (1834–99), medical officer of health for Marylebone and a teetotaller since the age of twenty-one, served as the SSI's first president and directed its agenda. He propounded the theory that habitual inebriety or dipsomania was a defect of the nervous system closely allied to insanity. The disease condition was usually caused either by a hereditary taint or by excessive indulgence itself, owing to alcohol's special affinity for brain cells. The 'depraved, debilitated, or defective nervous organisation' of the dipsomaniac was manifested as a morbid impulse for intoxication.[32] The exciting causes of inebriety were said to be located in the stressful conditions of modern life, with special reference to the experiences of the middle-class patients attended by Kerr and his colleagues on both sides of the Atlantic.[33]

These ideas were derived from the French alienist Bénédict Augustin Morel's (1809–73) theory of dégénérescence.[34] According to Morel, the hereditary diathesis (innate nervous defect) that gave rise to a tendency to alcoholism in one generation might have presented in the parents or ancestors as other diseases and disabilities. Kerr explained his use of the concept of degeneration and the phenomenon of transformation of heredity as follows: 'the inherited neuropathic predisposition may be transmitted, transformed into a variety of neurotic forms, the special form of insanity, inebriety, paralysis, epilepsy, hysteria, spasmodic asthma, hay fever, or allied nerve inheritance ...'.[35]

Kerr's extensive writings most clearly delineated the various meanings of 'inherited' inebriety in late nineteenth-century British medicine and social reform. Although ideas about hereditary causation and degeneration could have led to therapeutic nihilism, Kerr and the other SSI medical experts instead insisted that they had demonstrated the 'great truth that Inebriety is a disease, as curable as most other diseases, calling for medical, mental and moral treatment'.[36] They presumed that many, or even most, drunkards could be reclaimed if only they were provided with constant and long-term medical attention in an institutional setting. The short prison sentences customarily handed out to drunken offenders could do nothing to address the root of their problems: habitual drunkards were notorious as police court recidivists who, once released from prison, invariably returned to their dissolute ways. The disease concept of inebriety thus served both to account for this behaviour and to legitimise medical treatment.

In England, the 1879 Habitual Drunkards Act enabled the licensing and inspection of private 'retreats' for the *voluntary* admission of 'persons not subject to any jurisdiction in lunacy' whom two magistrates were willing to certify as in need of addiction treatment as 'a danger to himself, or herself, or to others, or incapable of managing himself or herself, or his or her affairs'.[37] Since the drunkard, or a sponsor, had to fully cover the costs of this care, 'the middle classes could afford treatment in retreats whilst there was no alternative other than to send working-class habitual drunkards without the means to pay the fees to prison'.[38] During the 1880s six such retreats were licensed serving eighty paying patients, and by 1910 there were twenty-five facilities in operation. Kerr and the SSI had urged that, in most cases, a one- to three-year term in a retreat would be sufficient time for a patient to cultivate the power of self-control and restore healthy nervous tissue. In actual practice, medical therapy for middle-class and wealthy drinkers consisted simply of withdrawal to one of these private retreats, or to a doctor's quiet country home, where the patient could enjoy a healthy diet, exercise and relaxation. The typical treatment regimen was ridiculed in *The Times* as amounting to 'a year of idleness under a course of Seltzer water and lemonade'.[39]

By contrast with their success in establishing a system of 'temporary refuge for gentleman alcoholics', the inebriety doctors at this time proved unsuccessful in lobbying the government to establish a parallel set of institutions for destitute habitual drunkards.[40] They were therefore disheartened by the Habitual Drunkards Act because it was limited to voluntary admissions (so as not to interfere with citizens' 'liberties') and because it did not extend to offering (compulsory) treatment for lower-class, criminal drunkards. Nonetheless, claims for the rehabilitation of 'affluent, self-declared drunkards' created career opportunities and professional respectability for the inebriety specialists, centred on a construct of organic mental disability.[41] The borderland disability of alcoholism further served the interests of patients themselves and their families.[42] Kerr and his colleagues published cases from their private practice in which families and friends affected by a drunkard's behaviour were relieved to be able to place him into treatment. Recognition of mental disability as the source of his troubles could bring access to at least a nominal form of healthcare, helping the drunkard to escape, as Kerr put it, from 'the finger of scorn ... pointed at the sot as an object of ridicule and contempt'.[43]

The disease concept of inebriety created an intermediate space where drunkenness could be defined as both medical and moral. As a borderland disability, it could be demarcated from religious and character-based approaches to the alcohol problem, while also maintaining culturally and legally valued notions that the drinker was culpable for his actions. Kerr explained that even though inebriates were victims of a physical, inherited condition and therefore should not be 'scorned', it was also necessary that these patients should learn to recognise their personal responsibility for their own recovery:

> It has been pleaded that to concede inebriety to be a physical disease will result in the inebriate believing that his conduct is beyond his control, that he is irresponsible for his inebriate indulgence, and that there is no chance of his deliverance from a career of drunkenness … So, far from riveting the chains of inebriety on the inheritor of the disease, a knowledge of his actual condition will indicate the adoption of such a regimen and mode of life as will promote health, as will decrease the morbid derangement while increasing the power of resistance and control.[44]

'Where to Get Men': racial deterioration and maternal drinking

By around 1900, a marked shift took place in the populations principally targeted by medical experts and social activists preoccupied with the 'vicious habit'. The Royal Commission on the Liquor Licensing Laws, which reported in 1899, turned the attention of physicians, politicians and the public towards the supposedly growing problem of working-class female drunkenness.[45] The Edwardian era thus saw the emergence of borderland configurations of disability around the figures of the female habitual drunkard and, more broadly, the unfit working-class mother. Although public anxieties about so-called racial degeneration were framed in the masculinising terms of military statistics and an industrial workforce, the problem of intemperance came to be 'feminized and domesticated'.[46]

'Where to Get Men' was the title of an influential 1902 article written by the British Army general Sir John Frederick Maurice (1841–1912), in which he observed that an alarming percentage of recruits were proving to be ineffective soldiers.[47] Concerns about where to get men who were physically and mentally fit for military service and other productive labour were echoed by prominent politicians such as the Liberal Imperialist leader Lord Rosebery (1847–1929), who urged in 1902 that medical knowledge be used to transform a 'drink-sodden population' into 'an Imperial race, a race vigorous, industrious and intrepid'.[48] Social Darwinists likewise argued that rising rates of crime and drunkenness in the slums meant that as many as half of the nation's unemployed were 'physically, mentally and morally unfit, [and so] there is nothing that the nation can do for these men except to let them die out by leaving them alone'.[49] This resurgence of degenerationist rhetoric fuelled the nascent British eugenics movement and led to official public health inquiries, including the Inter-Departmental Committee on Physical Deterioration.

The 1904 Physical Deterioration Report concluded that Great Britain's standing in the world was threatened by the deleterious effects of modern urban life on the bodies of people whom the expert witnesses labelled with such derogatory terms as 'unfit casual labour', 'wastrels' and 'rubbish'.[50] Urban overcrowding, inadequate diet and 'abuse of alcoholic stimulants' were found to be the leading causes of poor health in adults and of high infant morbidity and mortality. Testimony was provided by physicians and medical officers of health affiliated with the SSI and the National Temperance League, who framed inebriety as disease rather than vice. Another finding of the Report was that it would be more valuable to educate parents and children in the science of alcohol than 'expatiating on the moral wickedness of drinking'. The Report further emphasised how the increasing use of intoxicating beverages by poor and working-class women had 'consequences extremely prejudicial to the care of offspring, not to speak of the possibility of children being born permanently disabled'.[51]

As Gareth Stedman Jones has shown in his classic study *Outcast London*, at the time of the unemployment crisis of the 1890s, conversations about the condition of England emphasised the theory of urban degeneration as a biological rationalisation for the continued existence of extreme poverty and the risk of social unrest.[52] In this climate of anxieties about the urban lower classes, and especially women's responsibility for racial degeneration, intemperance became strongly associated with reproduction.[53] The 'new critique of alcohol' emphasised its racial and public health effects on women and children.[54] Working-class and poor women were now the principal targets of strategies to control inebriety, which involved control of the drink trade and of women's access to public houses, forced removal of habitual drunkards from society and maternal education. This contrasted sharply with the Victorian policies of supporting inebriates' retreats that offered idleness to affluent males in the guise of medical treatment.

After the turn of the century, authorities working within the administrative apparatuses of prisons, asylums and public health felt empowered to place more emphasis on society's right to restrict the liberty of drunkards, who already 'suffer an abatement of liberty' because of their diseased minds.[55] Compulsory confinement to a new system of inebriate reformatories went into effect in the period 1898 to 1913. To be identified as an inebriate with a criminal conviction meant risking exclusion from mainstream society for a sentence of one to three years in an institution 'whose mandate was on the border line between ... rehabilitation and punishment'.[56]

There were fourteen inebriate reformatories run by local authorities (financed by government and charitable donations) and two under the control of the Prison Commissioners. They housed a total of 4,600 convicted drunkards, mainly working-class and 80 per cent of them women.[57] Of the women in the reformatories, 400 had been accused of child neglect.[58] Proportionately, women were vastly overrepresented: 'in 1910, for example, out of a total of 143,708 [drunkenness] offences, 82 per cent (117,754) were committed by men.'[59] Most convicted male working-class drunkards instead served short prison terms, on the argument that they were the principal breadwinners and their families could not afford to lose them for a one- to three-year sentence in a reformatory.[60]

The treatment received inside the reformatories was more moral than medical, featuring total abstinence and traditional female chores such as cleaning, cooking, sewing and farm work.[61] Efforts to rehabilitate these unfit alcoholic mothers were therefore an extreme example of the educative impulse that characterised the Edwardian maternal and child welfare movement.[62] In practice, most of the 4,000 female inebriates came to be perceived by the reformatory managers as irredeemable: their alcoholism was diagnosed as a disability of either heritable feeble-mindedness or insanity, which caused their lack of self-control.[63] The perceived failure to more widely use the 1898 law, and the questionable outcomes of the treatment provided, led to the dismantling of the inebriate reformatory system by 1921.[64] After the passage of the 1913 Mental Deficiency Act, many lower-class female problem drinkers found themselves committed instead to custodial institutions for the feeble-minded as medical and administrative authorities readily altered their borderland classifications to adapt to the new legal landscape for social control.[65]

Medical experts in the SSI further advocated for the committal of inebriates even without criminal convictions, and for indeterminate sentencing. They argued in part that it was important to control the fertility of that 75 per cent of alcoholic women who were unmarried, separated from their husbands or believed to be prostitutes.[66] Thus the authorities did not hesitate to institutionalise, preferably for the duration of her reproductive years, both the socially useless alcoholic woman who had no family to care for and the married alcoholic woman whose family would be better off without her until she was cured of her addiction.

The problem of female intemperance was framed more widely than just the confinement of criminal alcoholic repeat offenders. Numerous witnesses to the 1899 Royal Commission on Liquor Licensing had highlighted the role of grocers' licenses in facilitating all working-class women's access to alcohol, while some temperance and inebriety physicians noted that *all* working-class families were spending too much of their wages on drink, and that even better-off women of the labouring classes were turning to drink to drown their problems.[67] Medical science explained that women's access to alcohol was a cause for alarm because women as a group were more susceptible to its deleterious effects than were men. Moreover, as historian Michelle McClellan argues, medical beliefs about middle-class female alcoholics hinged upon the attribution of disability to all women. The theory 'followed from the widespread belief that women's reproductive functions rendered them vulnerable to ill health, and that such alleged frailty could lead to reliance on medicine, including alcohol'.[68]

The meanings of alcoholism as disability were inflected by, and in turn served to shape, ideologies of gender at this time. For example, the inspector of the inebriate reformatories in 1909 described the weaker sex's vulnerabilities: 'A drunken woman nearly always becomes hysterical under the influence of drink ... Consequently, drunken women usually get into trouble.' The drunken man, by contrast, is 'inoffensive if left alone', although admittedly 'it is best to draw the curtain over what happens when he does get home'.[69] Thus, men's abusive behaviour lay outside the purview of scientific discussion, whereas working-class women effectively had inferiority or disability attributed to them. As a group, women were accused of risking the well-being of their families, for example by their supposedly documented tendencies to overlay their infants in bed and to neglect their child-care duties. Some writers even claimed that the non-drinking working-class housewife fostered the alcohol problem and thereby posed a threat to the family, society and the construct of masculinity:

> [She has] an appalling ignorance of everything connected with cookery, with cleanliness, with the management of children, [making her] one of the most helpless and thriftless of beings, and which therefore impels the workman, whose comfort depends on her, not only to spend his free time in the public house, but also tends to make him look to alcohol as a necessary condiment with his tasteless and indigestible diet.[70]

Conclusion: borders and intersections

This outline of shifting medical and administrative responses to inebriety in England illustrates sites where alcohol use factored into various configurations of disability, gender and class. Locating alcoholism as a kind of borderland disability also raises critical questions about the relationship between pathology and moral deviance in the history of disability. In the Victorian era, the discourses and practices around inebriety were focused on legitimising a concept of alcoholism that centred the drunkard who was truly 'deserving' of empathy and medical resources: he was a victim of hereditary disease. Physicians and legislators established provisions to support affluent drinkers towards recovery, rescue them from stigma and restore their middle-class male privileges. But the struggle to demarcate deserving from undeserving problem drinkers was never fully resolved.

Medical experts rhetorically distanced themselves from the 'partisan moralising' of the temperance movement, but at the same time they also conceded that mentally disabled inebriates should be held morally responsible for their vices: it was the patient's personal duty to avoid exposure to alcohol and to seek medical treatment when the craving 'overpowered the judgement and will'.[71] The medical profession, prior to 1900, also advocated for expansion of the inebriate institutions to include involuntary confinement of lower-class alcoholics, but the government refused to implement such expensive and invasive medical intervention for a much larger population. It was expected that lower-class male drinkers should be able to personally control their excesses through moral restraint, without recourse to any formal supports, or else end up in jail for short periods of time that would not excessively interfere with their gendered roles as breadwinners.

After 1900, physicians and policy makers adopted a new set of strategies for policing the boundary between the disease of alcoholism and the vice of drunkenness in order to satisfy a new set of agendas. Several thousand lower-class female drunkards were designated as mentally disabled to justify controlling their deviant behaviour and sexuality by means of removal and surveillance in the inebriate reformatories. An individual committed within that system may have been offered better support for some of her needs than ordinary criminal incarceration would have provided. At the same time, the poor and working-class women who were marked as drunkards but *not* subjected to forced removal to the reformatories were provided with even less support. It might be suggested that this too was a form of oppression, made possible at the borderlands of alcoholism where problem drinking was not officially recognised as pathological enough to qualify for significant intervention.

Much of the rhetoric of the Edwardian period around women's responsibility for racial degeneration marked all female bodies as inferior to male bodies, and therefore disabled, owing to their greater susceptibility to alcohol. All working-class women were also blamed for creating disability in their children through their 'personal failings' in the domestic sphere. Yet, despite these close linkages between female alcoholism and attributions of disability, these women whose drinking was considered socially and racially dangerous were effectively classified as not truly needy: not disabled enough to qualify for public assistance. Their deficiencies as mothers were blamed not on a diseased mind but instead on personal ignorance and incompetence; the borderland conditions of inebriety and imbecility both served to attribute to them moral failings as women and race mothers. Their situations involving real domestic and economic distress were disregarded and their demands for access to resources to better support themselves and their families were systematically denied. None of the Edwardian responses to the detrimental consequences of maternal drinking addressed the socio-economic and patriarchal roots of the problems that working-class women identified for themselves, such as overwork, low wages, lack of access to medical care and excessive childbearing.[72]

The ways that expert and public discourses patrolled the boundaries demarcating deserving from undeserving, and pathological from immoral, had varying effects on people's lives. Critical attention to borderland disability entities can help to uncover systems of power, including professional interests and social control, and to press us to think about the complexity of ongoing medical-scientific, policy and cultural confrontations with issues of alcohol use. At the borderlands we gain critical insight into 'the ways that classifications of defectives were influenced by issues of race, class and gender or how racial, class and gender concerns were in turn framed by novel approaches to mental and physical aptitude.'[73] The borderland between disability history and the medical history of inebriety and intemperance can also enrich our knowledge of disabled people's lives and complicate existing narratives about oppression and access to resources.

Notes

1 W. F. Bynum, 'Alcoholism and degeneration in 19th century European medicine and psychiatry', *British Journal of Addiction*, 79 (1984), 59–70.

2 D. Gutzke, '"The cry of the children": the Edwardian medical campaign against maternal drinking', *British Journal of Addiction*, 79 (1984), 71–84.

3 L. Radzinowicz and R. Hood, 'Curing and restricting the habitual drunkard', in L. Radzinowicz and R. Hood (eds), *A History of English Criminal Law and Its Administration from 1750*, vol. 5 (London: Stevens and Sons, 1986), pp. 288–315; R. MacLeod, 'The edge of hope: social policy and chronic alcoholism, 1870–1900', *Journal of the History of Medicine and Allied Sciences*, 22 (1967), 215–45.

4 G. Hunt, J. Mellor, and J. Turner, 'Wretched, hatless and miserably clad: women and the inebriate reformatories, 1900–1913', *British Journal of Sociology*, 40 (1989), 244–70.

5 J. Woiak, 'A medical Cromwell to depose King Alcohol: medical scientists, temperance reformers, and the alcohol problem in Britain', *Histoire Sociale/Social History*, 27 (1994), 337–65; P. McCandless, '"Curses of civilization": insanity and drunkenness in Victorian Britain', *British Journal of Addiction*, 79 (1984), 49–58; G. Johnstone, 'From vice to disease? The concepts of dipsomania and inebriety, 1860–1908', *Social and Legal Studies*, 5 (1996), 37–56; P. Carpenter, 'Missionaries with the hopeless? Inebriety, mental deficiency and the burdens', *British Journal of Learning Disabilities*, 28 (2000), 60–4; J. H. Warner, 'Physiological theory and therapeutic explanation in the 1860s: the British debate on the medical use of alcohol', *Bulletin of the History of Medicine*, 54 (1980), 235–57; G. W. Olsen, '"Physician heal thyself":

drink, temperance and the medical question in the Victorian and Edwardian church',
Addiction, 89:9 (1994), 1167–76.

6   W. F. Bynum, R. Warner and H. L. Rosett, 'The effects of drinking on offspring: an
historical survey of the American and British literature', *Journal of Studies on Alcohol*,
36 (1975), 1395–420.

7   H. Rimke and A. Hunt, 'From sinners to degenerates: the medicalization of morality
in the 19th century', *History of the Human Sciences*, 15 (2002), 59–88; M. Valverde,
'"Slavery from within": the invention of alcoholism and the question of free will',
Social History, 22 (1977), 251–68; A. Barton, '"Wayward girls and wicked women":
two centuries of "semi-penal" control', *Liverpool Law Review*, 22 (2000), 157–71;
C. May, 'Habitual drunkards and the invention of alcoholism: susceptibility
and culpability in nineteenth century medicine', *Addiction Research*, 5 (1997),
169–87.

8   J. Woiak, 'Drunkenness, Degeneration, and Eugenics in Britain, 1900–1914' (PhD
thesis, University of Toronto, 1998); Gutzke, 'Cry of the children'; J. Lewis, *The
Politics of Motherhood* (London: Croom Helm, 1980), pp. 61–88.

9   C. M. Crabbe, 'On the Borderland of Insanity: Women, Dipsomania and Inebriety,
1879–1913' (PhD thesis, University of the West of England, 2014); B. Morrison,
'Ordering Disorderly Women: Female Drunkenness in England c. 1870–1920'
(PhD thesis, Keele University, 2005); P. Carpenter, *A History of Brentry: House,
Reformatory, Colony and Hospital* (Bristol: Friends of Glenside Hospital Museum,
2002); P. McLaughlin, 'Inebriate reformatories in Scotland: an institutional history',
in S. Barrows and R. Room (eds), *Drinking: Behavior and Belief in Modern History*
(Berkeley, CA: University of California Press, 1991), pp. 287–314; D. Beckingham,
'An historical geography of liberty: Lancashire and the Inebriates Act', *Journal of
Historical Geography*, 36 (2010), 388–401.

10 M. Thomson, *The Problem of Mental Deficiency: Eugenics, Democracy, and Social
Policy in Britain, c. 1870–1959* (Sheffield: Clarendon, 1998), p. 22.

11 B. Linker, 'On the borderland of medical and disability history: a survey of the
fields', *Bulletin of the History of Medicine*, 87 (2013), 499–535.

12 M. Jackson, *The Borderland of Imbecility: Medicine, Society, and the Fabrication of
the Feeble Mind in Late Victorian and Edwardian England* (Manchester: Manchester
University Press, 2000), pp. 12–13.

13 *Ibid.*, pp. viii and 13.

14 *Ibid.*, pp. 7 and 3.

15 Crabbe, 'Borderland of Insanity', p. 2. Another key historiographical source Crabbe
cites for the concept of the borderland is E. Showalter, *The Female Malady: Women,
Madness, and English Culture, 1830–1980* (London: Virago, 1987), p. 106.

16 Crabbe, 'Borderland of Insanity', p. 4.

17 *Ibid.*, p. 101.

18 *Ibid.*, p. 24.

19 Jackson, *Borderland of Imbecility*, p. 13. Jackson cites in particular H. Maudsley,
Responsibility in Mental Disease (London: Henry S. King, 1874), and A. F. Tredgold,
Mental Deficiency (London: Bailliere, Tindall and Cox, 1908).

20 Woiak, 'A medical Cromwell'; on the British temperance movement generally, B. Harrison, *Drink and the Victorians: The Temperance Question in England, 1815–1872* (London: Faber and Faber, 1971).

21 Maudsley, *Responsibility in Mental Disease*.

22 B. Gilbert, 'Health and politics: the British Physical Deterioration Report', *Bulletin of the History of Medicine*, 39 (1965), 143–53; R. A. Soloway, 'Counting the degenerates: the statistics of race deterioration in Edwardian England', *Journal of Contemporary History*, 17 (1982), 137–64.

23 Crabbe, 'Borderland of Insanity', pp. 22–3.

24 A. Borsay, *Disability and Social Policy in Britain since 1750: A History of Exclusion* (Basingstoke: Palgrave Macmillan, 2005), pp. 11–12; quoting from D. Stone, *The Disabled State* (Philadelphia, PA: Temple University Press, 1984).

25 On the British idiot asylums as welfare provisions, see D. Wright, *Mental Disability in Victorian England: The Earlswood Asylum, 1847–1901* (Oxford: Clarendon, 2001); on alcoholism, deviance and the welfare state in the United States, see J. Gusfield, *Contested Meanings: The Construction of Alcohol Problems* (Madison, WI: University of Wisconsin Press, 1996).

26 Jackson, *Borderland of Imbecility*, p. 13.

27 W. B. Carpenter, *On the Use and Abuse of Alcoholic Liquors in Health and Disease* (Boston, MA: Crosby and Nichols, 1851), pp. 39–41; R. B. Grindrod, *Bacchus, An Essay on the Nature, Causes, Effects, and Cure of Intemperance* (Hartford, CT: S. Andrus and Sons, 1851), pp. 290–2; B. Richardson, *Ten Lectures on Alcohol* (New York, NY: National Temperance Society, 1887), p. 177.

28 E. Parsons, *Manhood Lost: Fallen Drunkards and Redeeming Women in the Nineteenth-century United States* (Baltimore, MD: Johns Hopkins University Press, 2003).

29 Harrison, *Drink and the Victorians*, pp. 127–33; L. L. Shiman, *Crusade Against Drink in Victorian England* (New York, NY: St Martin's, 1988), pp. 23–4, 29–33.

30 V. Berridge, 'The Society for the Study of Addiction: 1884–1988', *British Journal of Addiction*, 85 (1990), 983–1087; L. Blumberg, 'The American Association for the Study and Cure of Inebriety', *Alcoholism: Clinical and Experimental Research*, 2 (1978), 235–40; E. M. Brown, 'English interests in the treatment of alcoholism in the US during the early 1870s', *British Journal of Addiction*, 81 (1986), 545–51; S. Tracy, *Alcoholism in America: From Reconstruction to Prohibition* (Baltimore, MD: Johns Hopkins University Press, 2005).

31 N. Kerr, *Inebriety, or Narcomania: Its Etiology, Pathology, Treatment and Jurisprudence*, 3rd edn (London: H. K. Lewis, 1894), p. 198.

32 N. Kerr, 'President's inaugural address', *Proceedings of the Society for the Study of Inebriety*, 1 (1884), 3.

33 M. Rotunda, 'Savages to the left of me, neurasthenics to the right, stuck in the middle with you: inebriety and human nature in American society, 1855–1900', *Canadian Bulletin of the History of Medicine*, 24 (2007), 49–65.

34 B. A. Morel, *Traité des dégénérescences physiques, intellectuelles et morales de l'espèce humaine* (Paris: J. B. Baillière, 1857); D. Pick, *Faces of degeneration: A European disorder, c. 1848–c. 1918* (Cambridge: Cambridge University Press, 1989).

35   Kerr, *Inebriety*, p. 36.

36   *Ibid.*, p. xii.

37   MacLeod, 'The edge of hope'; J. Nicholls, *The Politics of Alcohol: A History of the Drink Question in England* (Manchester: Manchester University Press, 2009).

38   Crabbe, 'Borderland of Insanity', pp. 43–4.

39   Quoted in Radzinowicz and Hood, 'Curing and restricting', p. 299.

40   *Ibid.*, pp. 294–300.

41   Berridge, 'Society for the Study of Addiction', 999.

42   On complex family motivations for institutionalisation, see Wright, *Mental Disability*, p. 8.

43   Kerr, *Inebriety*, p. 3.

44   *Ibid.*, p. 17. He elsewhere argued against alcoholics' criminal responsibility, by analogy with the insanity defence. N. Kerr, 'Inebriate criminal responsibility', *Proceedings of the Society for the Study of Inebriety*, 16 (1888), 12–14.

45   D. Wright and C. Chorniawry, 'Women and drink in Edwardian England', *Canadian Historical Association's Historical Papers* (1985), 118–19.

46   V. Heggie, 'Lies, damn lies, and Manchester's recruiting statistics: degeneration as an "urban legend" in Victorian and Edwardian Britain', *Journal of the History of Medicine and Allied Sciences*, 63 (2008), 178–216.

47   Sir J. F. Maurice, 'Where to get men', *Contemporary Review*, 81 (1902), 78–86.

48   Lord Rosebery, *Miscellanies, Literary and Historical* (London: Hodder and Stoughton, 1921).

49   A. White, 'The nomad poor of London', *Contemporary Review*, 47 (1885), 714–27, quoted in G. S. Jones, *Outcast London: A Study in the Relationship between Classes in Victorian Society* (New York, NY: Pantheon, 1984), pp. 288–9.

50   G. R. Searle, *The Quest for National Efficiency: A Study in British Politics and British Political Thought, 1899–1914* (Oxford: Blackwell, 1971).

51   *Report of the Inter-Departmental Committee on Physical Deterioration, Parliamentary Papers*, XXXII.1–780 (HMSO, 1904), Vol. 1, pp. xxxii, 1, 5, 13 and 31. The inebriety and temperance doctors' testimony was published in Vol. 3, pp. 721–9; see also Gutzke, 'Cry of the children', 73–4.

52   Jones, *Outcast London*, pp. 283–7. See, for example, J. Cantlie, *Degeneration amongst Londoners* (1885; New York, NY: Garland 1985).

53   In his 1894 book, *Inebriety*, Norman Kerr made only passing references to supposed impairments in the children of intemperate parents, pp. 192 and 718. The topic of heredity became much more prominent in SSI writings after 1900, starting with 'Report of the Committee on Heredity', *Proceedings of the Society for the Study of Inebriety*, 68 (1901), 1–12.

54   Gutzke, 'Cry of the children', 71. Some examples from the time period include R. Parr, 'Alcoholism and cruelty to children', *British Journal of Inebriety*, 6 (1908), 77–81; S. Atkinson, 'Care of children neglected by drunken parents', in National Conference on Infantile Mortality, *Report of the Proceedings of the National Conference on Infantile Mortality: Held in the Caxton Hall, Westminster, on the 23rd, 24th, and 25th*

March 1908 (London: P. S. King & Son, 1908), pp. 146–71; F. Zanetti, 'Inebriety in women and its influence on child life', *British Journal of Inebriety*, 1 (1903), 47–57; E. W. Hope, 'Infant mortality as affected by the habits of the parents', in National Conference on Infantile Mortality, *Report of the Proceedings of the National Conference on Infantile Mortality: Held in the Caxton Hall, Westminster, on the 23rd, 24th, and 25th March 1908* (London: P. S. King & Son, 1908), 139–45.

55   W. C. Sullivan, 'The criminal responsibility of the alcoholic', *British Journal of Inebriety*, 2 (1904), 53.

56   Hunt *et al.*, 'Wretched, hatless and miserably clad', 245.

57   Radzinowicz and Hood, 'Curing and restricting', pp. 301–15; L. Zedner, *Women, Crime and Custody in Victorian England* (Oxford: Oxford University Press, 1991).

58   Hunt *et al.*, 'Wretched, hatless and miserably clad', 247.

59   *Ibid.*, 246.

60   *Ibid.*, 258; Morrison, 'Ordering Disorderly Women', pp. 253–60.

61   Hunt *et al.*, 'Wretched, hatless and miserably clad', 259–60; Morrison, 'Ordering Disorderly Women', pp. 263–311 fully examines the disciplinary regimes and agency experienced by women in the Langho reformatory; M. McClellan, 'Historical perspectives on alcoholism treatment for women in the United States, 1870–1990', *Alcoholism Treatment Quarterly*, 29 (2011), 332–56.

62   Morrison, 'Ordering Disorderly Women', p. 275–9; A. Davin, 'Imperialism and motherhood', *History Workshop: A Journal of Socialist Historians*, 5 (1978), 9–65; D. Dwork, *War Is Good for Babies and other Young Children: A History of the Infant and Child Welfare Movement in England 1898–1918* (London: Tavistock, 1987).

63   Hunt *et al.*, 'Wretched, hatless and miserably clad', 250–1.

64   Radzinowicz and Hood, 'Curing and restricting', p. 314.

65   Jackson, *Borderland of Imbecility*, pp. 201–26 on the Mental Deficiency Act.

66   Hunt *et al.*, 'Wretched, hatless and miserably clad', 250–1.

67   Wright and Chorniawry, 'Women and drink', 127–8.

68   McClellan, 'Historical perspectives', 334–5.

69   R. W. Branthwaite, *The Report of the Inspector under the Inebriates Acts, for the Year 1909, Parliamentary Papers*, XXIX.11 (HMSO, 1911), p. 27.

70   W. C. Sullivan, *Alcoholism: A Chapter in Social Pathology* (James Nisbet, 1906), p. 111.

71   J. Parrish, 1872 address to the American Association for the Cure of Inebriety, quoted in Tracy, *Alcoholism in America*, p. 30; McClellan, 'Historical perspectives', 333; Berridge, 'Society for the Study of Addiction,' 997; McCandless, 'Curses of civilization', 53–4.

72   Women's Co-operative Guild, *Maternity: Letters from Working-Women* (London: G. Bell, 1915; reprint Garland, 1980).

73   Jackson, *Borderland of Imbecility*, p. 7.

6

VICTORIAN MEDICAL AWARENESS OF CHILDHOOD LANGUAGE DISABILITIES

Paula Hellal and Marjorie Lorch

From the mid-nineteenth century, disability in childhood became an issue of increasing interest to the British medical and educational communities as 'Victorians sought to better identify, categorise and manage those individuals who were unable to conform to society's expectations'.[1] With the founding of the first paediatric hospitals and the introduction of compulsory elementary education, children's abilities and disabilities were analysed and assessed on an unprecedented scale. Many of the children admitted to the new specialist hospitals had chronic debilitating conditions, necessitating their treatment on the wards or in convalescent homes for extended periods. This provided the opportunity for physicians to follow up on the progress of their young patients and conduct longitudinal studies of their recovery.

Beginning in the 1860s, there were several decades of research into the significance of acquired disorders of language in previously healthy adults. However, it was not until the end of the century that clinicians began to focus their attention on children who failed to develop speech or learn how to read. This new medical interest in children with language disabilities was driven by the social concern of parents and educators and by the clinical appreciation of the maturational trajectory for the neurological organisation of language. In this chapter we will explore Victorian attitudes to childhood disability by focusing on how physicians attempted to describe and explain these newly identified developmental disorders of language.

The scientific study of children

Some tradition of providing institutional support for those with sensory impairments already existed in early modern Britain at the beginning of the nineteenth century. The first public school for the education of deaf individuals opened in London in 1792, with more schools following the capital's lead: Liverpool, Manchester, Exeter and Doncaster all opened establishments in the 1820s. A school for blind people opened in Liverpool in 1791, and that too was followed by others opening around the country, for example, Edinburgh, Bristol, London and Norwich had asylums for blind children (and adults) by the beginning of the nineteenth century.[2] By mid-century, a school for 'physically handicapped' girls had opened in London, with a similar institution for boys opening in the following decade. Around this time, in response to social, economic and political pressures, on the one hand, and medical and scientific agendas, on the other, a growing number of state schools and charitable institutions started to offer some training and education to children with physical or sensory impairment.

However, it was not until the latter part of the century that the sheer number of children affected with some sort of disability became apparent. The turning point was the 1870 and 1880 Education Acts, which made elementary education compulsory in England for all under the age of thirteen.[3] During the nineteenth century the population of Britain had increased dramatically, and by the time the 1870 Act came into effect it had reached twenty-six million, with more than three million inhabitants in London alone. Children from deprived urban areas began to enter school for the first time and the appalling scale of poverty, sickness and mental and physical impairments was no longer hidden.

Almost immediately, there were growing calls for welfare provision. In an attempt to discover how serious the problem was, the British Medical Association, the Charity Organisation Society and the British Association for the Advancement of Science set up a committee in 1888 with the objective to conduct a study into the development of 100,000 school children. Its report, edited by Francis Galton (1822–1911), included recommendations on the type of education and training that would be most suited for 'handicapped' children.[4] In 1893 the Elementary Education (Blind and Deaf Children) Act, which established special schools for those with sensory impairments, was passed; and in 1899 the Elementary Education (Defective and Epileptic Children) Act made the same provision for physically impaired children.[5]

It was not only within the educational domain that disabled children were examined, assessed and trained.[6] This period also saw new specialist paediatric hospitals founded across the country, although throughout much of the nineteenth century British medical opinion proved stubbornly opposed to any type of specialisation. Providing separate medical facilities for children was particularly anathema to many.[7] The common concern was that a sick child would fail to thrive if taken from its mother, while allowing mothers to remain with their children in the hospital would, it was thought, cause the spread of infection.

Among the few who thought otherwise was Dr Charles West (1816–98). West had trained on the continent of Europe, where children's hospitals were already established. The first was L'Hôpital des Enfants Malades, which was founded in Paris for children under the age of fifteen years in 1802. In 1821 the Institute for Sick Children was founded in Dublin, and in the 1830s specialist paediatric hospital provision was created in Berlin, St Petersburg, Vienna and Breslau.[8] By the 1840s, West had returned to England and was working at the Universal Dispensary in Waterloo Road, London, the only institution in the capital that provided out-patient care for mothers and infants. West was keen to establish a paediatric hospital. That there was a pressing need for such an institution is made clear in a contemporary report criticising the lack of provision for the treatment of the diseases of children:

> neither in this city [London] nor throughout the whole British empire is there any hospital exclusively devoted to their reception. At the same time, the number of children received into the general hospitals is so small, that on an enumeration of the population of those institutions, made in January 1843 … they were found to contain only 136 children under 10 years of age. Of this small number … only 26 [had been admitted] for the cure of any internal disease.[9]

In the same year, and after a lengthy struggle, West founded the Hospital for Sick Children in Great Ormond Street, London. Other paediatric establishments soon followed, with hospitals opening in several cities across Britain, including in Norwich (1853), Manchester (1855), Edinburgh (1860) and Birmingham (1861). A second London hospital, the Evelina, was established in 1869, through the personal generosity of Ferdinand de Rothschild (1839–98), to provide for sick children who lived south of the River Thames. By the turn of the century, more than twenty-five paediatric hospitals had been established in towns and cities across Great Britain, and there were also specialist institutions, such as the Alexandra Hospital for Hip Disease in London, which cared exclusively for children with congenital musculoskeletal afflictions.

Children were frequently kept as in-patients in the paediatric hospitals for months on end. For example, in the Evelina Hospital the average length of stay in 1876 was sixty days.[10] This long-stay care arrangement may in part have been due to the lack of adequate home support and the general social deprivation of these young patients. Home conditions were often recorded in the Great Ormond Street patient case notes, for example, as being 'poor' or 'unsatisfactory'. Furthermore, it was common practice for hospital staff to arrange for recuperating children to stay at a convalescent home, usually located in the countryside or at the seaside, for a period of time after being discharged. This ensured that they had good food, fresh air, rest and ongoing medical attention that was typically lacking in their home environment, while at the same time freeing the limited number of hospital beds for more acutely ill patients. The number of these convalescent homes had been growing in England and Wales from the 1860s, and by the last decade of the century there were about fifty. Some were independent institutions that contracted beds out to the city hospitals, while others belonged to the urban paediatric hospitals. In 1869 Great Ormond Street Hospital leased its own convalescent home for sick children, Cromwell House in Highbury, which was then a small village four miles outside the city of London.

The importance of age as a factor in disease

As Charles West had hoped, the establishment of the children's hospitals led to a rapid increase in research into childhood disease. Clinical observations from large numbers of children began to be collated and compared. It became apparent that an important variable was the age of the patient at symptom onset. This understanding enabled physicians to investigate new questions and draw original distinctions between perinatal, infant and later childhood illness.[11] These distinctions were most evident in the investigations of infantile cerebral paralysis and acquired childhood aphasia.[12]

John William Little (1810–94) was the first to draw significant attention to the developmental difficulties of children with infantile cerebral paralysis, examining the condition initially from an orthopaedic point of view.[13] Physicians caring for large numbers of children in the new hospitals began to publish case series in an attempt to differentiate infantile cerebral paralysis from paralysis due to spinal lesions. William Osler (1849–1919), who popularised the use of the term 'cerebral palsy', presented a case series highlighting the relevance of the age of the child when their symptoms began to the diagnosis and prognosis of their condition.[14] Osler also pointed out that the effects of cerebral palsy extended beyond difficulties with motor control and general mental development, to particular consequences for the development of language.

Language impairment

The neurological underpinnings of speech impairment were brought to medical attention by the French physician Paul Broca (1824–80), who, in the 1860s, suggested a link between impaired language function and damage in the frontal cortex found at autopsy.[15] Following his reports, numerous case studies started to appear in the literature. Children were typically reported alongside adults without comment.

Tracing these case studies poses specific challenges at different points of time throughout the nineteenth century. There is the watershed moment when the French term '*aphasie*' was coined in 1864,[16] but before this time, and indeed for some further period following, such symptoms were most likely to be recorded in English hospital patient records and medical publications as 'loss of speech' or 'speechlessness'. In such cases an individual's language would have been developing typically (or at least without apparent difficulty) before a brain injury of some description resulted in noticeable difficulty with speech.

It was only towards the end of the century, when the syndrome was already a well-established clinical entity, that the link was made between the age of the patient at the time when the brain injury occurred and the severity of symptoms, patterns of recovery and likelihood of lasting deficits in language.[17] This parallels the attention being paid to age at symptom onset in the emerging clinical category of cerebral palsy. Cases of children who had been acquiring language in a typical fashion until illness or trauma resulted in loss or impairment were, by their nature, relatively rare. Far more common were instances of children who failed to develop language normally. However, until the last decade of the nineteenth century, these children were conspicuous by their absence from hospital records and the published medical literature. Until the 1890s, children with developmental language difficulties might have found themselves in asylums for the 'feeble minded' or, if they were fortunate, they might have had some remedial help from specialists in the education of deaf people or even from elocution masters. Also at this time, difficulties in the development of related language abilities such as reading and writing began to be noted by physicians rather than by educationalists.

Terminology

In these late nineteenth-century observations, symptomatic behaviour was described in detail. However, no clear terminology or classificatory system had yet been developed. In contrast to the syndrome of aphasia, which was a well-recognised clinical entity by 1870, the developmental disorders of language or related selective cognitive difficulties did not enter the accepted nosology until a century later. The term 'congenital word-blindness' was used for many decades to describe the developmental reading difficulties which are today referred to as 'dyslexia'. This term, along with the broader concept of 'learning disability', was not introduced until the 1960s.[18]

The social historians Risse and Warner point out that, in order to understand its social and medical meaning, a diagnosis must be placed within a contemporary classification system.[19] Medical labels have been defined and redefined over time. In the field of developmental language impairments, including reading difficulties, there have been a multiplicity of labels used to describe the same condition. In their review of the literature from the mid-nineteenth century onwards, Worster-Drought and Allen commented on the plethora of terms used:

> The history of the subject of congenital word-deafness and its complications is a reflection of the different phases through which the subject has passed since aphasia was first recognised as a clinical abnormality early in the nineteenth century. Hence it follows that references to the subject are to be found under the headings of idiocy in children, speech defects (and especially idioglossia), congenital aphasia, sensory aphasia, congenital word-deafness, the association of congenital word-deafness and congenital aphasia with speech defects, behaviour defects, studies in psychology and educational problems.[20]

Their view draws on evidence taken from a wide range of monographs, textbooks and medical journal articles covering a period of more than fifty years.

The descriptions of such behavioural symptoms were generally brief, including only a few sentences concerned with medical history, physical appearance, general demeanour and the nature of the child's understanding and production of speech.[21] At the same time, the selectivity of the cases represented in the medical literature must be acknowledged. The motivation for publishing cases illustrating particular disabilities varied; for example, to establish the existence of a particular symptom, address a contemporaneous theoretical debate, illustrate an unusual reaction to standard treatment or demonstrate a successful new treatment.

Dyslexia

Initial interest in impaired literacy during the mid-nineteenth century focused on the underlying relation of impairments in spoken and written expression. The theoretical question at stake was whether an individual with a difficulty in producing speech could, or could not, write. Up until the 1880s there was an assumption that both spoken and written production relied upon the language faculty and could not be selectively affected by a cortical brain lesion that preserved speech.[22] This concern with writing may also have reflected the more selective social status of this attainment at the time. In the eighteenth and early nineteenth centuries, wide ranges of individuals from various social backgrounds were taught to read, often in a domestic setting, for the sole purpose of reading the Bible.[23] However, this practice did not represent true functional literacy for such individuals. As Victorian plans for universal education were realised, a greater number of children learned not only to read but also to write, in a formal school setting. Finally, towards the turn to the twentieth century, concerns about children with such difficulties began to become evident. Anderson and Meier-Hedde make the point that:

> Of all the early research that was devoted to dyslexia, the work that was accomplished in the United Kingdom during this time period … became enormously significant for several reasons. First, the United Kingdom physicians wrote with a clarity and organization that heretofore had not been observed in the literature. Second, they turned attention to the plight of children, and, third, these physicians wrote numerous case reports on word blindness, which resulted in an accumulation of information about this enigma. A virtual explosion of research came out of the United Kingdom in the early twentieth century. Previous research had been sporadic, in part because researchers had not specialized in this disorder. The United Kingdom physicians investigated reading problems as a primary research interest, which enabled them to make a greater contribution in this area … The early case reports of the United Kingdom physicians would have continuing influence on all work that would come later.[24]

William Pringle Morgan (1861–1934) reported one of the earliest cases of developmental reading difficulties in a child in an 1896 issue of the medical journal *The Lancet*. Morgan was a general practitioner who also delivered medical services to the nearby preparatory schools in Sussex. He described fourteen-year-old Percy K, who had 'always been a bright and intelligent boy', was noted to be 'quick at games, and in no way inferior to others of his age', but who never learned to read.[25] Morgan suggested by analogy to the pattern found in acute acquired disorders of reading that the boy's 'visual word centre' had failed to develop normally. This hypothesis was a developmental extension of psychophysical models of brain localisations for particular cognitive functions that had been developed to explain adult acquired difficulties with language processes with respect to the auditory, visual and motor modalities.[26]

Morgan admitted that his notice of this case was prompted by the description, the year before, of acquired reading difficulties in adults by James Hinshelwood (1859–1919): 'My reason for publishing this case was that there was no reference anywhere, so far as I knew, to the possibility of this condition being congenital.'[27] There was immediate interest in the appearance of reading difficulties in children following Morgan's case description, with more than two dozen papers on the topic appearing in the first decade of the twentieth century.[28] Hinshelwood began to see increasing numbers of children who had failed to learn how to read at his ophthalmological clinic, and published an influential series of papers on childhood reading disability based on a large series of cases between 1895 and 1911.[29]

Developmental language disorder

Like developmental dyslexia, developmental language disorder was only described decades after the adult-acquired counterpart. In the early 1890s a series of papers were published detailing the cases of children whose speech had failed to develop in a typical fashion. Walter Bough Hadden (1856–93), a young physician at Great Ormond Street Hospital, brought his first such case to the attention of the medical community in 1891. Hadden described an otherwise healthy child who was treated for a lengthy period as a hospital in-patient for his lack of progress in language acquisition. The boy had an extreme defect of articulation, although there was no mechanical difficulty. He could not utter any sounds until he was three or four years old, and as he grew older could still not produce even words of one syllable in an intelligible fashion.[30] Hadden drew an initial analogy between the development of walking and speech; both needed special muscular coordination, and would therefore show variation in developmental rates. He proposed that treatment for such speech disabilities must be informed by details of typical language development.

Shortly following this report, other London clinicians presented similar cases.[31] A nine-year-old boy was brought to St Thomas' Hospital for advice. His schoolmistress found the child's speech incomprehensible and proposed that he should be sent to the Deaf and Dumb Asylum. The clinicians determined that the boy was not deaf and set about treating his articulation difficulties.[32] These early reports, describing otherwise healthy children admitted to hospital for developmental language impairment, mark the start of modern research into the condition.[33]

Studying child language acquisition

By the latter decades of the nineteenth century, physicians had a number of motives for considering the acquisition of language in the child. As we have seen above, they hoped that an understanding of the process would illuminate abnormal development. There was also another consideration: it was generally held that adult aphasics re-acquired speech in much the same manner as a child learned to talk. Therefore, it was suggested that understanding how children proceed to learn language might assist in the development of remedial therapy for aphasic adults. Within the medical literature the stages of language acquisition in the child were typically described by reference to research into localisation of function in the brain and observations of acquired aphasia.[34]

The initial stage was thought to involve the child learning to associate sounds with particular objects. Medical textbooks of the time describe the infant being taught this recognition directly by the mother uttering a word while pointing to the relevant object.[35] It was hypothesised that the association between utterance and object would become fixed in the child's auditory speech centre by means of repetition. The development of the motor centre would allow the child to reproduce the words heard.

However, it was not only physicians who were interested in child language acquisition. By the latter half of the nineteenth century child development had become a new subject of empirical research by psychologists and educators with particular interest in language. While the increasing focus on child development was generally coincident with social, economic and political developments in Victorian Britain, there was an academic motivation as well. These early psychologists considered the emerging complexity of children's behaviour as relevant to the Darwinian theory of human evolution.

Observations of Charles Darwin's (1809–82) own son, recorded in his personal diary in the 1830s, served as the basis for what is typically viewed as the first English publication on infant development.[36] The paper by Darwin, a scientist of international renown, attracted widespread attention. English psychologist-fathers were inspired to publish scholarly reports on their own infants' language development. This was a topic that previously was considered to belong firmly to the domestic domain of the nursery.[37] Although literate women had been keeping private diaries of their children's sayings and doings throughout the century and earlier, they were typically not publicly disseminated. This was true even of those written by otherwise respected and published novelists such as Elizabeth Gaskell (1810–65).

In one further respect, parents contributed to the growing interest in child language acquisition and disorders. They took their concerns that their child was 'late in talking' to their physician for advice. In order to respond to this complaint in a clinical context, physicians needed to have a norm against which they could compare their young patient. Determination of what constituted delayed language development was drawn from evidence in reports from the growing paediatric clinics in hospitals and the burgeoning diary studies by the psychologists. The general view of physicians was that, where there was no indication of disease or deformity, and a child could hear and seemed 'bright', speech might be merely delayed in development. However, they had very little besides their own judgement to bring to the task of determining a child's mental abilities when speech was not an avenue for assessment.

As West pointed out, 'a child's inability to describe its sensations deprives us of another important guide'.[38] The child's previous history was also seen as a potential diagnostic aid. However, the difficulty of obtaining an accurate medical history was compounded in a number of cases by the onset of presenting symptoms occurring before (in many cases a long time before) the child was seen by a physician. The all-important early history of a condition, vital for accurate diagnosis, was typically acquired at second hand, the informant in most cases being the child's mother.

The medical educator Francis Warner (1847–1926) offered advice in his textbook on conducting the medical examination of a child:

> It is convenient to commence with some general conversation on simple subjects – e.g., his life at school or at home, in play and at work; what he reads, his companions and amusements. The faculty of speech is thus ascertained and some idea of the extent of his vocabulary. Various defects of speech may be found; there may be ill regulated intonation, the voice at times almost dying away; there may be thickness of utterance, often in part due to nasal-pharyngeal obstruction; a few words may be spoken in reply to a question without affording an answer; the question may simply be repeated without any reply. In many other particulars speech or utterance may be defective. ... Particularly notice in conversation whether the child makes comparisons or exercises the faculty of judgement ... The behaviour of the child with common objects may show much as to his modes of dealing with his surroundings ... In children with little or no speech it is more difficult to ascertain whether a judgement is formed.[39]

As well as assessing the language-delayed child's mental capabilities, clinicians appreciated that deafness had to be ruled out first as a contributing factor. West, decades earlier, had commented on how difficult it was to determine the existence of congenital deafness in early childhood.[40] As deafness could be partial, assessment was complicated and physicians might erroneously label the child as intellectually deficient. West had also seen cases where difficulty of articulation, perhaps partly dependent on malformation of the mouth, had resulted in similarly inappropriate classification. However, by the 1890s significant advances had been made and assessment of developmental language impairment was beginning to be put on a scientific footing, enabling comparison between cases.

As mentioned above, before the end of the nineteenth century many children who failed to develop language normally were assumed to have a general impairment in mental ability or auditory perception. Some were placed in institutes for the deaf or asylums for imbeciles, and, as a consequence, would not receive adequate schooling. This was despite the fact that many patients with developmental language difficulties were described as 'intelligent'. Well into the twentieth century, some institutions for the education of mutes would not admit or even examine children who could hear and were mute, or had very little speech, as it was thought that their condition was hopeless and they were unsuitable for any type of education.[41]

Remediation

In the late nineteenth century the only group that typically received therapeutic intervention was deaf-mutes. Little had been developed by this point to assist in the recovery of adults with acquired language impairments. In the case of children with acquired language disorders, remedial measures were not considered necessary as it was a widely held medical opinion that these children would swiftly recover their language abilities. However, the growing interest in developmental language disorders led to attempts to devise treatment regimes, some involving intensive one-to-one remediation with specialist staff over long periods.

The Scottish physician John Wyllie (1844–1916) employed a child's father to treat his son's developmental language disorder by means of 'the physiological alphabet'. Wyllie initially described such an approach with reference to an adult aphasic case:

> We did not trouble the patient with the names of the letters, but taught him from the beginning the letter-sounds of the physiological alphabet. In doing so, we adopted what may be called the 'Mother's Method'. Beginning with the Labials, we taught him to say papa, apap, appa, thus giving him the consonant P as an initial, a terminal and a mid-letter … and so on throughout the alphabet. He was shown by 'lip-reading' how to place the lips, tongue, etc., for the pronunciation of each letter-sound.[42]

Hadden, in contrast, made use of the Oral Method that originated in Germany in his efforts in speech remediation. The method had been established in some London schools for deaf children from the late 1860s.[43] The practice directed the teacher to face the pupil and show, by exaggerated movements of his own lips and tongue, the positions to form each particular sound. Sight and touch were used in place of the defective sense of hearing.[44] Hadden used this method to treat a boy hospitalised for seven weeks. At the end of this remediation period, Hadden noted that the boy could successfully produce individual letter names, but had a repertoire of only a few simple words and phrases. However, Ashby and Wright point out that successful treatment of defective speech depended on the cause of the condition. The mother of another patient of Hadden's was trained in the Oral Method for the deaf and attended the treatment sessions between the nurse and her child at the hospital.

Involving parents in therapy for childhood speech disorders was an innovation that was less practised as speech and language therapy became a fully fledged profession in the mid-twentieth century. Possible therapies for word blindness were also being put forward only a few years later. At the turn of the century, Hinshelwood recommended strengthening sight–sound association for children afflicted with word blindness through the use of touch. He proposed using block letters that the child could feel as well as see to assist in overcoming reading difficulties.[45]

In general, longitudinal descriptions of an individual's pattern of recovery were rarely reported in the medical literature as cases were typically published shortly after the child's admission to hospital. Moreover, often in the nineteenth century, once a patient had left the hospital there was little or no follow-up care. However, some Victorian paediatricians made great efforts to follow up their patients' progress, observing the children's development or lack thereof over periods of months and sometimes years. Their work led, from the last decade of the nineteenth century, to attempts being made to formalise assessment procedures and to improve and develop speech transcription methods. Hale-White and Golding-Bird even made use of the recently invented phonograph to make recordings (now lost) of their patients' pre- and post-treatment speech samples.[46]

Although individual clinicians had developed their own investigative procedures, these methods were yet to be widely adopted and standardised.[47] Linguistic science, upon which a rigorous understanding of language is based, was still in its infancy, although in the latter part of the century books on phonetics and grammar were beginning to appear. Throughout the century, the Victorian physician had to rely on his own, and his colleagues', clinical judgement and experience when presented with cases of impaired language function. Their descriptions of linguistic impairments were, therefore, somewhat idiosyncratic. Given that the clinical examination of grammatical aspects of language was very rudimentary even in adult aphasia until later in the twentieth century, it is unsurprising that the assessment and remediation of speech difficulties in children focused almost entirely on the phonetic analysis of speech.

Conclusions

During the Victorian period a new focus on childhood disabilities of language developed. Hospitals, asylums, schools and specialist establishments were opened throughout Britain. There were growing efforts to systematically describe the prevalence, cause, prognosis and treatment of such disabilities, although, as Starkey points out, 'if the experiences of physically disabled children can be said to have improved by the end of the century ... children afflicted with epilepsy or mental health difficulties were less likely to benefit from greater understanding'.[48]

Initially, children were served by the same social and medical systems as adults. However, as the century progressed, it became increasingly common to consider the needs of children separately from issues that concerned the adult population: Acts of Parliament focusing on childhood issues were passed; paediatric hospitals treated childhood disease and assessed child development. There was a steady increase in specialist terminology and models of developmental language disabilities, while the patient's age at the onset of symptoms came to be recognised as a relevant determining clinical factor in the compromise of speech and literacy.

The nineteenth-century interest in child language acquisition was initiated in England by Charles Darwin, with larger-scale group studies following throughout the latter decades of the century, such as psychologist James Sully's (1842–1923) *Studies of Childhood*.[49] As well as the publication of individual patient reports, medical textbooks began to describe both developmental and acquired language disorders in childhood, such as language delay, stammering, stuttering and aphasia. This increased interest within the medical profession, in typical and deviant child language acquisition, made it possible for physicians to begin to compare their patients' language development with the perceived standard. Conditions now termed developmental dysarthria, specific language impairment and dyslexia were investigated around this time. As the first papers on such disorders started to appear, many physicians realised that they too had seen similar cases. This is a specific instance of the general experience that once a new phenomenon is formally identified, it is subsequently found to be surprisingly common. Investigations of language disabilities grew in number following the publication and discussion of the first few cases. Many research-ers, both in Britain and abroad, followed the work of these early Victorian pioneers.

At the turn of the twentieth century child development and, in particular, child language disorders were being studied on a large scale both in the English-speaking world and on the Continent by those involved in medicine, psychology, education and social welfare. By examining this early period of research into childhood language disorders we can trace the development of contemporary concerns and debates. The late Victorians were interested in many of the same questions that we are preoccupied with today: what constitutes language delay? What can be done to assist children with delayed or impaired speech? And why do some children struggle to read or pay attention? The Victorian era can be credited with ushering in reforms in any number of important areas concerning disabilities, from childhood developmental disorders, including, but not limited to, problems with language acquisition, to mental health issues that affected both young and old. These early steps in recognising age as a factor of clinical importance were responsible, in large part, for eventual legislation in Great Britain, continental Europe and the United States that provided equitable treatment of children and adults alike.

Notes

1   A. R. Rosenthal, 'Insanity, family and community in late-Victorian Britain', in A. Borsay and P. Dale (eds), *Disabled Children: Contested Caring 1850–1979* (London: Pickering and Chatto, 2012), pp. 29–42, at p. 29.

2   D. Gillard, *Education in England: A Brief History* (2011), available online at www.educationengland.org.uk/history/.

3   Compulsory education for children aged between five and thirteen was introduced in Scotland by the Education (Scotland) Act of 1872.

4   D. S. Galton, *Report on the Scientific Study of the Mental and Physical Conditions of Childhood, with Particular Reference to Children of Defective Constitution: And with Recommendations as to Education and Training*, Committee on the Mental and Physical Condition of Children (London: British Medical Association, 1895).

5   The 1893 Act for England and Wales was preceded in Scotland by the 1890 Education of Blind and Deaf-Mute Children (Scotland) Act.

6   A. Turmel, *A Historical Sociology of Childhood* (Cambridge: Cambridge University Press, 2008).

7   W. F. Bynum, *Science and the Practice of Medicine in the Nineteenth Century* (Cambridge: Cambridge University Press, 1994).

8   A. Ballabriga, 'One century of paediatrics in Europe', in B. L. Nichols, A. Ballabriga and N. Kretchmer (eds), *History of Paediatrics 1850–1950* (New York, NY: Raven Press Ltd, 1991).

9   R. Ellis, *Diseases in Childhood* (London: G. Cox, 1852), p. 8.

10 E. Lomax, 'Small and special: the development of hospitals for children in Victorian Britain', *Medical History*, Supplement No. 16 (1996).

11 For example, see H. C. Bastian, *On Paralysis from Brain Damage in Its Common Forms* (London: Macmillan, 1875); W. Osler, *The Cerebral Palsies of Children. A Clinical Study from the Infirmary for Nervous Diseases*, reprinted edition, Vol. 1, Classics in Developmental Medicine 1 (Philadelphia, PA: Mac Keith Press, 1889; reprinted 1987); S. Freud, *Infantile Cerebral Paralysis [Die Infantile Cerebrallähmung]*, trans. L. A. Russin (Miami, FL: University of Miami Press, 1897).

12 P. Hellal and M. Lorch, 'Darwin's contribution to the study of child development and language acquisition', *Language & History*, 53:1 (2010), 1–14.

13 W. J. Little, 'Hospital for the cure of deformities: course of lectures on the deformities of the human frame', *The Lancet*, 41:1053 (1843), 350–4.

14 Osler, *Cerebral Palsies*.

15 P. Broca, 'Perte de la parole, ramollissement chronique et destruction partielle du lobe antérieur gauche du cerveau', *Bulletins de la Société d'anthropologie*, 2 (1861), 235–8; 'Du siège de la faculté du langage articulé dans l'hémisphère gauche du cerveau', *Bulletins de la Société d'anthropologie*, 6:6 (1865), 377–93; 'Nouvelle observation d'aphémie produite par une lésion de la troisième circonvolution frontale', *Bulletins de la Société d'Anatomie (Paris)*, 6 (1861), 398–407.

16 Armand Trousseau, 'De l'aphasie, maladie d'écrite recomment sous le nom impropre d'aphémie', *Gazette des Hôpitaux Civils et Militaires*, 1 (1864), 13–14.

17 For example, see W. Elder, *Aphasia and the Cerebral Speech Mechanism* (London: H. K. Lewis, 1897); J. Ross, *On Aphasia: Being a Contribution to the Subject of the Dissolution of Speech from Cerebral Disease* (London: J. and A. Churchill, 1887); J. Wyllie, *The Disorders of Speech* (Edinburgh: Oliver and Boyd, 1894).

18 D. Hallahan and W. Cruickshank, *Psychoeducational Foundations of Learning Disabilities* (Englewood Cliffs, NJ: Prentice-Hall, 1973).

19 G. Risse and J. Warner, 'Reconstructing clinical activities: patient records in medical history', *Social History of Medicine*, 5:2 (1992), 182–203.

20 C. Worster-Drought and I. M. Allen, 'Congenital auditory imperception (congenital word-deafness): and its relation to idioglossia and other speech defects', *Journal of Neurology and Psychopathology*, 10:39 (1930), 193–236, at 196.

21 P. S. Weiner, 'The study of childhood language disorders: nineteenth century perspectives', *Journal of Communication Disorders*, 19:1 (1986), 1–47.

22 M. Lorch, 'The history of written language disorders: re-examining Pitres' case (1884) of pure agraphia', *Brain and Language*, 85:2 (2003), 271–9.

23 T. Thornton, *Handwriting in America: A Cultural History* (New Haven, CT: Yale University Press, 1996).

24 P. L. Anderson and R. Meier-Hedde, 'Early case reports of dyslexia in the United States and Europe', *Journal of Learning Disabilities*, 34:1 (2001), 9–21, at 12.

25 W. P. Morgan, 'A case of congenital word-blindness', *British Medical Journal*, 2:1871 (1896), 1378.

26 For example, see H. C. Bastian, 'On the various forms of loss of speech in cerebral disease', *British and Foreign Medical-Chirurgical Review*, 43 (1869), 209–36, 470–92.

27 W. M. H. Behan, 'James Hinshelwood (1859–1919) and developmental dyslexia', in F. C. Rose (ed.), *Twentieth Century Neurology: The British Contribution* (London: Imperial College Press, 2001), pp. 59–76, at p. 60.

28 For example, see E. Nettleship, 'Cases of congenital word-blindness (inability to learn to read)', *Ophthalmic Review*, 20 (1901), 61–7; J. H. Fisher, 'Case of congenital word-blindness (inability to learn to read)', *Ophthalmic Review*, 24 (1905), 315–18; A. L. Benton, *Exploring the History of Neuropsychology: Selected Papers* (Oxford: Oxford University Press, 2000).

29 Behan, 'James Hinshelwood'.

30 W. B. Hadden, 'On certain defects of articulation in children, with cases illustrating the results of education on the oral system', *Journal of Mental Science*, 37 (1891), 96–105.

31 For example, see W. H. White and C. H. Golding-Bird, 'Two cases of idioglossia with phonographic demonstration of the peculiarity of speech', *Transactions of the Medical and Chirurgical Society*, 74 (1891), 181–9; F. Taylor, 'A case of defective articulation', *Transactions of the Medical and Chirurgical Society*, 74 (1891), 191–7.

32 White and Golding-Bird, 'Two cases of idioglossia'.

33 M. Lorch and P. Hellal, 'The "idioglossia" cases of the 1890s and the clinical investigation and treatment of developmental language impairment', *Cortex*, 48:8 (2012), 1052–60.

34 For example, see B. Bramwell, 'Lectures on aphasia', *Edinburgh Medical Journal*, 11 (1897), 1–13, 117–28, 232–45, 356–70, 454–65, 527–51.

35 *Ibid.*

36 C. Darwin, 'Biographical sketch of an infant', *Mind*, 2:7 (1877), 285–94.

37 M. Lorch and P. Hellal, 'Darwin's "natural science of babies"', *Journal of the History of the Neurosciences*, 19 (2010), 140–57.

38 C. West, *Lectures on the Diseases of Infancy and Childhood* (London: Longman, Brown, Green and Longmans, 1884), p. 242.

39 F. Warner, 'Neural and mental disorder in children', in W. Edwards (ed.), *Cyclopedia of the Diseases of Children; Medical and Surgical, Recent Literature. Volume 5, Supplement* (Philadelphia, PA: J. B. Lippincott Co, 1899), pp. 1304–16, at p. 1311.

40 C. West, *On Some Disorders of the Nervous System in Childhood*, Lumleian Lectures. (London: Longmans, Green and Co, 1871); West, *Lectures on the Diseases of Infancy and Childhood*.

41 T. Barlow, 'On a case of double hemiplegia, with cerebral symmetrical lesions', *The British Medical Journal*, 2 (1877), 103–4. This case is discussed in P. Hellal and M. Lorch, 'Discrepancies between the published and archived case notes of the most cited case of acquired child aphasia in the 19th century', *Journal of the History of the Neurosciences*, 16 (2007), 378–94; White and Golding-Bird, 'Two cases of idioglossia'.

42 Wyllie, *The Disorders of Speech*, p. 327.

43 J. Ree, *I See a Voice: Language, Deafness and the Senses – a Philosophical History* (London: Harper Collins, 1999).

44 H. Ashby and G. Wright, *The Diseases of Children* (London: Longmans, 1892).

45 J. Hinshelwood, *Letter-, Word- and Mind-Blindness* (London: H. K. Lewis, 1900).

46 Anonymous, 'The phonograph in medicine', *British Medical Journal*, 1:1575 (1891), 537.

47 L. S. Jacyna, *Lost Words: Narratives of Language and the Brain 1825–1926* (Princeton, NJ: Princeton University Press, 2000); M. Lorch 'Examining language functions: a reassessment of Bastian's contribution to aphasia assessment', *Brain*, 136:8 (2013), 2629–37.

48 P. Starkey, 'Club feet and charity: children at the House of Charity, Soho, 1848–1914', in A. Borsay and P. Dale (eds), *Disabled Children: Contested Caring 1850–1979* (London: Pickering and Chatto, 2012), pp. 15–28, at p. 27.

49 J. Sully, *Studies of Childhood* (London: Longmans, Green, and Co, 1895).

7

'HAPPINESS AND USEFULNESS INCREASED': CONSUMING ABILITY IN THE ANTEBELLUM ARTIFICIAL LIMB MARKET

Caroline Lieffers

In the winter of 1845–46 a young man from New Hampshire, auspiciously named Benjamin Franklin Palmer (c. 1824–98), carefully carved a piece of willow into the shape of a leg.[1] Inside, he fitted a complex apparatus for coordinated flexion and extension of the knee, ankle and toes. The following November, Palmer was granted the first patent for a prosthetic limb in the United States, and soon the 'Palmer Patent Leg' dominated the mid-nineteenth-century prosthesis market.[2]

Palmer is a key figure in the history of disability and prostheses, but his early career remains relatively unexamined by historians. The most significant studies of American artificial limbs have focused on the period after the Civil War (1861–65), viewing the rehabilitated, industrialised body as an essential symbol for a nation in recovery, ravaged by conflict and flooded with perhaps 45,000 amputation survivors.[3] Palmer had a central role in this postbellum market, but as early as 1857, four years before the opening salvo at Fort Sumter, he estimated that nearly 3,000 of his limbs were already in use.[4]

This chapter begins with a survey of Palmer's personal and business history. Focusing on the antebellum period, it argues that the enterprising manufacturer was already successfully marketing a brand of innovative triumph over medicalised disability well before the outbreak of war. This marketing took place in a rapidly changing American nation, where industrial capitalism and technological innovation led to increased manufactures, exports and urbanisation – and the emergence of stigmatised categories of disability among people who did not readily conform to these new patterns of work.[5] In this heady commercial arena, the artificial limb was presented as a desirable consumer product, sold under the seductive and prestigious banner of science and technology. As depicted in Palmer's promotional literature, amputation and prostheses were not signs of weakness, but opportunities for the products of American innovation to surmount medical and social challenges.

The second half of this chapter traces the alleged effects of Palmer's celebrated appliance on Americans' lives – at least, as presented in the manufacturer's advertisements, reviews and testimonials. Although the reported names, locations and occupations of these ostensibly enthusiastic limb wearers generally correspond with census records, the testimonials were likely solicited. The dates of the letters, moreover, were often changed to make the accounts seem more current, and consistency of style and diction suggests that these supposedly personal narratives were heavily edited. But the testimonial genre, which even in the nineteenth century would not have been completely credible, highlights the artificial limb's discursive place in antebellum culture and hints, to some extent at least, at users' feelings about, and experiences with, their prostheses.[6] These first-hand accounts, however suspect, enumerate the uses, both rhetorical and practical, to which the artificial limb and the mobility it facilitated might be put. The prosthesis, wearers suggested, was able to merge with the body, making them feel 'whole' again, physically and mentally, and it could facilitate masculine ideals of sociability, labour and business success. Indeed, despite a steady presence of women in Palmer's promotional literature, men and masculinity were the default identities for artificial limb advertising, intimately connecting the appliance to a world of nineteenth-century male work, independence and sociability.

Disability activists and historians have pointed to the pre-eminence of what is now termed the 'medical model' of disability in the nineteenth century. This model, in contrast to models that emphasise societal barriers, treated bodily difference as an individual flaw or deficiency and looked to medical experts for its mitigation.[7] As the first half of this chapter points out, the Palmer limb drew much of its authority from medical approval. But the onus of inclusion in Palmer's advertising literature was always on the individual's material consumption. The medical model, I argue, was also a consumer model, in which bodily difference was imagined as open to intervention and resolution not only by medical professionals, but also by consumer products, the entrepreneurs willing to develop them, the surgeons willing to recommend them and the well-off people willing to buy them. Appealing to medical elites and popular desires alike, the Palmer limb demonstrates how bodily difference was looped into and shaped by the capitalist structures of medicine, entrepreneurial activity and consumer satisfaction.

Medicine and mechanism: the entrepreneur and the artificial limb

Between 1821 and 1846 accidents accounted for roughly one third of amputations at a hospital in urban Boston.[8] This was Palmer's own experience when, as a child growing up in New Hampshire, his leg was amputated following a mill accident. However, Palmer carried on. Promotional materials described him as a studious, virtuous and sociable young adult who published poems, taught writing and studied law. Still, '[f]eeling his misfortunate keenly', as one 1854 biography put it, he purchased a version of the Anglesey Leg, the prosthetic device famously supplied to Henry William Paget (1786–1854), Britain's earl of Uxbridge and later marquess of Anglesey, after he lost a leg at Waterloo.[9]

Palmer reportedly found the limb awkward, so he decided to try making his own. He developed mechanisms for better springiness and control, flexibility, durability and lightness, as well as minimal noise and more realistic colour, texture and shape, with nearly seamless joints. In May 1846 he exhibited this new leg in Washington, DC, where it reportedly met with acclaim, and he returned home to open a small shop in Meredith Bridge, New Hampshire.[10] In 1849 he relocated to the bustling city of Springfield, Massachusetts, and went into partnership with surgeon Erasmus Darwin Hudson (1805–80) and a series of artisans. Business was good and, as he continued to patent improvements to the leg, Palmer opened stores in Philadelphia and New York and moved his Springfield shop to even busier Boston. He distributed models of his invention to hospitals across the north-eastern United States and presented it at dozens of exhibitions; by 1856 it had garnered at least thirty awards.[11]

A wide-ranging promotional campaign was key to Palmer's success. His tale of self-reliance had democratic appeal; in 1853 a travel article in the *New York Daily Times* highlighted the town where he invented his leg, rising from 'poor lame boy' to great inventor.[12] Moreover, as a wearer of his prosthesis, Palmer was literally a walking testimonial. Articles emphasised his smooth gait – no one would suspect anything but a 'sound natural limb' – and clients validated Palmer on the basis of his personal experience.[13] One testimonial confirmed that 'after witnessing the remarkable degree of *ease, grace,* and *naturalness* with which you [Palmer] were enabled to walk upon one of your own Artificial limbs, we speedily procured one for my use'.[14]

Palmer did not stop at popular appeal. Indeed, he occupied the middle of what Paul Starr has called a 'dialectic between professionalism and the nation's democratic culture' in nineteenth-century American medicine.[15] In addition to being an inventor and problem-solver in the best democratic tradition, Palmer, without any formal medical training, cunningly enmeshed himself and his product in the values of medical science and expertise in order to construct an exclusive and desirable professional identity. Formerly, artificial legs might have been made by any number of craftsmen. Palmer, however, argued that the work of a skilled 'surgeon-artist', as he termed himself, was a crucial complement to surgery.[16] He explained that he and his partners had studied works of anatomy, surgery, mechanics and chemistry, and visited medical schools, hospitals and scientific institutions. Endorsements from prominent surgeons Henry Bigelow (1818–90) and Valentine Mott (1785–1865), along with technological associations and industrial award committees, preceded and often outnumbered those from patients in Palmer's brochures and advertisements, even in sectarian medical publications such as the *Water-Cure Journal*.[17] As Palmer put it, '[t]he Scientific Surgeon who skillfully removes the obnoxious limb, and the competent Surgeon-Artist who successfully replaces the same artistically, should be regarded as filling offices of coördinate [sic] importance, and each should be the colleague of the other'.[18] While his rivals and precursors were simply 'incompetent Artisans almost entirely ignorant of Anatomy, and even the laws of mechanics', Palmer stressed that his 'harmonious blending' of surgical science and subsidiary art secured 'the future happiness of the patient'.[19]

Aiming for professional parity, Palmer projected even the most mechanical aspects of the prosthesis through the prism of medical authority. Using anatomical vocabulary, Palmer and Hudson described the challenge of replicating 'inanimate bones, muscles, tendons, and cuticles', and they referred to the appliance's parts in terms of the Achilles tendon, flexors and extensors, and the ginglymoid hinge-joints of the knee and toes.[20] Medical and industrial societies apparently saw this sophisticated analogy to human anatomy as the essential reason for the leg's life-like functioning and seamless integration with the body; the appliance was 'a mechanical compensation of lost parts', as one exhibition jury put it.[21] While earlier limbs were noisy and required a halting stride, the Palmer leg was quiet, fluid and responsive. What was once a matter of a local craftsman's potentially unreliable skill had now become the pinnacle of American technological ingenuity, and patients and surgeons alike owed 'the highest obligation to the mechanic arts', to quote one write-up.[22]

At the same time, the leg's aesthetic appeal, with its attractive, hand-crafted exterior and customised socket, precluded any potential anxieties that might have accompanied technology's growing invasion into nineteenth-century daily life. This was no satanic mill or unsettling railway; each limb was custom-designed and custom-fitted, despite its mechanical components. And the Palmer leg was also meant to be consumed. At London's Great Exhibition in 1851, for example, the limb was featured in the American display and praised for its cosmetic elegance; although grounded in the category of 'Surgical Instruments', it was the pinnacle of technological and artistic achievement alike. Indeed, the Great

Exhibition has been described as an outburst of commodity culture and modern merchandising, where goods were worshipped above the 'mundane act of exchange'.[23] In this context, not only was the Palmer leg framed as a thing of beauty, but the prominent surgeons who served on the Exhibition's jury elevated and purified capitalistic competition by giving awards to the best products; Palmer earned a coveted prize medal.[24] This was as an object to be admired, revered and even coveted as art, not simply as machine or medical apparatus.

Exhibitions were also business opportunities, and, in Palmer's case, the product's success and surprising elegance ensured that it would be publicised well beyond its narrow clientele. *Punch* dedicated an article to the limb and joked that it could help posh families attain perfectly matching footmen for their carriages, while society ladies self-conscious about the shape of their legs might 'remedy the defects of nature by having recourse to this admirable American artist'.[25] The *New York Daily Times* and *The Times* of London also celebrated the product less satirically, suggesting at least some level of public comfort with amputation, especially when projected through the accepted lens of middle- and upper-class consumption, technological advancement and effective medical intervention.[26]

With his evocative name and appealing story of ingenuity, self-reliance and pursuant success, Palmer was a model citizen. National pride, too, figured prominently in the literature surrounding his invention. American journals recounted his European tour, documenting Yankee victory at every turn as Palmer conquered the professional, social and commercial worlds with unassuming American ease. He spoke to surgeons at the Hôtel-Dieu in Paris and was introduced 'as a conspicuous guest' at a party for 400 people at the Royal College of Surgeons in London. An unidentified Member of Parliament even 'proposed a walking match between English and American legs', and the latter reportedly won, earning Palmer 'the sobriquet of Anglesey junior'. The Maryland Institute reportedly toasted that 'the conquerors of Waterloo cannot walk without at least one Yankee leg'.[27]

The prosthesis also resuscitated the Americans' reputation at the Great Exhibition. The display had started badly for the United States, as they had brought too few items for the space they had reserved, and their focus on agricultural and natural products seemed coarse in comparison to other countries' statuary and silks.[28] But, with the help of the artificial limb, Palmer wrote, 'the London Times has frankly and manfully declared that the yankees [sic] "have taken the shine out of them," and has made the most ample reparation for all it said disparagingly of our representation in the Crystal Palace during the early part of the exhibition'.[29] Indeed, *The Times* reported that 'the artificial leg patented by Mr. Palmer, is, in its way, a most admirable, ingenious and philanthropic contrivance, and its invention is so remarkably characteristic of the country from whence it comes, that we cannot resist the temptation of inviting attention to it'. Palmer, like a 'true American', had sought to improve on earlier, unsatisfactory products.[30] According to Charles Stansbury, an organiser of the American display who later acted as Palmer's patent attorney, the nation owed 'a debt of gratitude' to men like Palmer, who 'so nobly vindicated the industrial honor of our country'.[31] Rather than drawing attention to the apparent problem of America's diseased and injured men and women, the limb was emblematic of an American solution and secured the country's place as a leading manufacturer of consumer goods. Ingenuity and improvement, even in fields as seemingly unusual as the manufacture of artificial limbs, found fruition in what commentators depicted as the democratic and industrialising United States. Palmer himself wrote:

> The present is an age of *inventions* and *exhibitions*. The International Exhibition in London was an epoch in history which disclosed the sinews of power in the arm of the useful arts. The inventor and the artisan were then, for the first time, duly honored, and their *rights* fully conceded. The anatomical mechanician has received all the honors to which his works entitle him, and we think more.[32]

Palmer had commanded diverse forms of authority, from emotional to medical to mechanical, and he presented a product that seemed to appeal to and exemplify the best and most exciting features and developments of its era. One client marvelled at the 'power of man to make and attach to me any thing so near nature'.[33] Although the United States – and Britain, for that matter – was flooded with new and desirable products, the 'American limb' seemed to satisfy contemporary commentator Alexis de Tocqueville's evocative ideal of a 'virtuous materialism' that would 'not corrupt, but enervate the soul, and noiselessly unbend its springs of action'.[34]

Fashion and function: the limb and its wearers

Palmer was poised to take advantage of an evolving consumer environment in the United States, and even further afield. Railways allowed more Americans to travel to the nearest Palmer & Co location for a fitting, or to have the artificial limb shipped to them. In a national market, branding became a crucial commercial tool, especially when competitors and counterfeiters emerged in the 1850s. Palmer vociferously attacked rivals who he believed compromised his reputation or infringed on his patents, including his former employees Darwin DeForrest Douglass and Benjamin W. Jewett. He warned that '[w]orkmen who were unable to manufacture the limb in such manner as to gain our confidence, because of their inefficiency, or lack of integrity, have the temerity to urge upon the unfortunate their clumsy imitations of our limbs as *improvements* or *original inventions*.[35] Even before the Civil War crowded the field with a wave of new patents and manufacturers, Palmer rightly assumed a nationally competitive business in which he needed to ensure an exclusive stake.

Urbanisation, too, altered the retail landscape. Palmer's offices were located in popular shopping districts, including Philadelphia's Chestnut Street and New York's Broadway, which one contemporary writer described as 'the most showy, the most crowded, and the richest fashionable thoroughfare on the continent'.[36] As Broadway developed into a stylish centre, the artificial limb – priced as high as a daunting $150, but often discounted for the lower classes – was not simply a medical apparatus but also an extension of the wardrobe. In London, Palmer even licensed his appliance to a firm on Savile Row, a street that was already attracting tailors and dealers in luxury goods.[37] What his literature called 'patients' thus found themselves in an experience that was as much commercial as medical. While the middle classes generally received medical treatment privately at home, the Palmer experience was meant to feel sociable, smart and genteel, and clients received obsequious service. Although, ideally, the artificial limb should not make itself known, if a man was spotted patronising Palmer's establishment he could be sure that he was associated with an expensive and sophisticated product, and he might be proud of having a leg that was conspicuously inconspicuous.

Perhaps most importantly, the limb contributed to the normalising goals of social conformity and participation. Although the limb might never be seen, its elegant and life-like appearance, 'covered with parchment, painted a flesh color and beautifully enameled', imparted confident carriage for the upwardly mobile.[38] Its 'perfect naturalness and high finish' took 'away all repulsiveness in its appearance', as one of Palmer's promotional articles put it, as well as 'the limping gait, and the unpleasant noise' that gave away other prostheses.[39] As Stephen Mihm has argued, physical appearance that affirmed the status of the self-made man was essential in a period in which social roles and identities were fluid and often suspect.[40] Fear of self-betrayal disciplined Americans who subscribed to regimens of work, exercise, temperance, grooming and comportment to affirm their positions. The role of the prosthesis in securing an impression of agency and gentlemanly self-government was clear in one of Palmer's early engravings (Figure 7.1), an expensive addition to his advertising materials that emphasised the appliance's social function. It featured six 'gentlemen', each missing both legs, whom Palmer counted as successful wearers of his products. Assuming dignified postures, complete with elegant suits and top hats, the men appear commanding and authoritative, their artificial limbs taking on a seamless corporeal shape beneath their impossibly absent lower trouser legs.

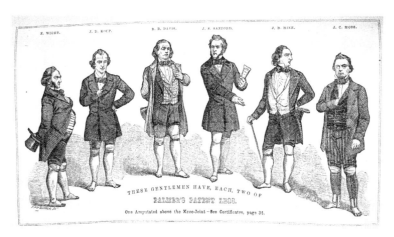

7.1 Illustration for Palmer's patent legs. Reproduced by permission of the National Library of Medicine, US Department of Health and Human Services.

Palmer himself also exemplified the success that could result from this kind of confident performance. Energetic and charming, he was elected vice-president of the New Hampshire Temperance Society, and a later brochure celebrated his horseback ascent of Mount Washington, accompanied by two friends.[41] Such social achievement might be read as an example of his missing leg's irrelevance in these contexts. Palmer, in fact, often portrayed himself as an inventor and a citizen first, highlighting his professional rather than personal knowledge of artificial limbs. In another analysis, however, Palmer's social performance was an extension of his walking testimonial. The prosthesis was always present, but revealed only when dramatically appropriate. '[A]fter walking some distance with Mr Palmer', wrote Alfred Velpeau's guide to surgery, 'we did not in the least suspect that he had himself been provided with one of his own artificial limbs, yet such is the fact, his leg having been amputated below the knee. It certainly is one of the greatest triumphs of American ingenuity.'[42] In granting the limb their top prize, Philadelphia's Franklin Institute similarly gushed that 'Mr Palmer, who has lost his leg just below the knee joint … is enabled, by means of his invention, to walk without a cane, in such a manner as readily to deceive one not acquainted with the facts of the case.'[43] Palmer went beyond simply 'passing' to avoid stigma: to dissemble and subsequently surprise observers heightened the achievement of 'conquering' disability with this new technology.[44]

The repeated emphasis on the confident gait that this limb facilitated also testifies to the centrality of posture and mobility as apparent measures of human dignity and independence. Artificial limbs forced an upright stance, a valuable position in an era in which rigid posture signified poise and class, and slouching or bending might imply primitivism, weakness or even femininity. As an advisor on physical carriage later in the century stated, '[a]ll those splendidly sexed always carry their shoulders well back and up'.[45] Stansbury observed that crutches often led to 'a long train of cruel sufferings', including problems with breathing, the nervous system and circulation.[46] Like the structured clothing of the period, the artificial limb was designed to create a proper figure as a sign of manliness, and its presence disciplined the whole physical and emotional system.[47] Walking, moreover, was central to gentlemanly leisure and socialising, and the conspicuously genteel streets on which Palmer had his shops were key sites of public life.[48] A later conduct book concurred that '[n]ot only is a man's walk an index of his character and of the grade of his culture, but it is also an index of the frame of mind he is in'.[49] Control of one's body and countenance signified agency and gentlemanly self-government, and Palmer occasionally included descriptions of men reduced to what he portrayed as the most abject condition, walking on their knees or all but dumped at his doorstep. He repeatedly featured J. S. Sanford, for example, a double amputee who 'was carried to Springfield, and placed on the floor before them [Messrs Palmer & Co] in a helpless condition. In a month's time he returned to his friends, with two as good appearing and acting limbs (apparently) as he ever had.'[50] Another patient, Matthew Palmer, was at first similarly 'weak and trembling, not having fully recovered from the shock of the accident and operation, and had had a pair of legs adjusted to his stumps [for] only three days; and yet it was marvelous, the ease and naturalness with which he walked about the house'.[51] Strapped on at the earliest possible moment, the devices seemed to restore the man almost instantly.

In their analyses of nineteenth-century artificial limbs, both Erin O'Connor and Lisa Herschbach stress the value of bodily wholeness for Victorian masculinity. As Herschbach expresses it, '[t]he aesthetics of prosthesis *mattered* because the artificial limb had to recover the man morally as well as physically'.[52] Stansbury, appealing for an extension to Palmer's patent just before the opening of the Civil War, might have concurred:

> 'A sound mind in a sound body,' is the comprehensive description of the state of a perfect man. The loss of a faculty, or of a member, destroys that enviable perfection; and to restore the one, or provide an adequate substitute for the other, is an object worthy of the highest efforts of beneficence.[53]

The prosthesis did not deceive. Rather, it restored men to an ideal of personhood. Stansbury equated the limb with the individual's mental faculty and reinforced the parallel by noting the 'moral' damage of limb loss, including 'mortified and wounded sensibilities'.[54] As one of Palmer's patients confirmed, 'I am now, thanks to your unequaled skill, enabled to move again in the society of my friends, to attend to my business, and, in short, I am *made whole*'.[55] Conflating physical, emotional and social meanings of wholeness, the writer testified to the object's psychic and relational work. The advertisements even implied that the limb's lightness and comfortable socket may have allowed wearers to forget their own amputations. In deeply inhabiting their prostheses, men could achieve a civility and an autonomy that penetrated and benefited their whole selves, public and private.

Although Palmer fought his way into the ranks of the medically respected, his product allowed the client to remove himself from the pathologised and passive world of medicine and reinsert himself into the independent, active arena of consumption, as well as production. Rosemarie Garland-Thomson has astutely argued that '[n]owhere is the disabled figure more troubling to American ideology and history than in relation to the concept of work: the system of production and distribution of economic resources in which the abstract principles of self-government, self-determination, autonomy, and progress are manifest most completely'.[56] The Palmer leg resolved disability's apparently rude violation of American norms and priorities, allowing '*mutilated individuals to walk erect as their fellow mortals*, and conceal the nature of their misfortune, as they engage in active and useful occupations'.[57] The *Boston Medical and Surgical Journal* similarly cheered that Palmer's patients might have their 'happiness and usefulness increased by being able to appear and act like perfectly-organized persons'.[58]

Many testimonials drew special attention to patients' capacity to do physical jobs. James McEleney, missing both legs, insisted that he would not be able to earn a living without his Palmer legs. With them, though, he could 'chop wood, use a pick, a spade, a saw, or do almost anything except hard laborious work'.[59] Another wrote:

> I can walk from three to five miles at one time with but little inconvenience. I generally have my limb in constant use from 8 o'clock A.M. until 11 o'clock P.M. in the store; and I find my stump feels much better while standing on my limb, than while sitting with or without the limb, as it seems to remove that twitching nervous affection that always attends an amputated limb.[60]

The pain of what physician Silas Weir Mitchell would later term a 'phantom limb' is reduced in this depiction to the agitations of the unproductive American.[61] Even professionals, who would not necessarily have needed the prosthesis for their labour, emphasised the product's functionality. A banker, for instance, wrote that '[t]he external appearance of your leg, may be judged of by any superficial observer. The real *beauty*, however, of an artificial leg to the unfortunate wearer, lies in its *utility*.'[62]

Indeed, in 1844 the Reverend Calvin Colton famously called America 'a country of *self-made men*', where 'work is held in the highest respect ... and the idle, lazy poor man gets little pity in his poverty'.[63] While *Scientific American* reviewed the leg for its mechanical interest, the article's introduction stressed its social function: 'instead of being at the mercy of their fellow-men for fresh air and exercise ... there are many who can attend to business, and thus make their livelihood'. They would otherwise have been 'helpless cripples – a trouble to their friends, and a burden to themselves all their lives'.[64] While the home and family had been the locus of care for generations of Americans who experienced the almost unavoidable reality of illness or injury, Palmer's patients expressed a new and sometimes extreme horror of dependency.[65] One declared that '[i]nstead of absolute helplessness and dependence, I am able to take my place in the active affairs of life, [and] contribute my full share to the accomplishment of its duties'.[66] Although in 1860 Stansbury claimed that '[w]e can never reduce the value of an invention like this, to exact pecuniary statement, until we learn to measure human sensibilities with a rule, and weigh human joys and sorrows in a balance', the attorney did not hesitate to calculate that, conservatively, the leg might have saved perhaps 500 Americans from charity at a cost of $500 each per year.[67] Providing a material remedy for disability was also an investment in the nation, obviating the risk of moral indolence and financial costs not only to individuals or their families, but also to society. Men who had lost their limbs in railway yards and factories now had an apparent obligation to return to work for the literal engines of American mobility and industry, beneficiaries rather than victims of technology's potential.

This sense of reversibility, the promise that a 'lost' limb might be 'found' again, entirely restoring the body and rescuing a person from the abhorrent state of familial or social dependency, often stretched into a seeming ambivalence about amputation, which came to distinguish limb loss from other forms of bodily difference.[68] As one review put it, '[t]his invention will obviate to a great degree the dread of amputation ... by creating the assurance that they [patients] can have their loss well nigh restored'.[69] The prosthesis was no garish appliance; that it did not need oil reinforced that it was more man than machine. One wearer testified that '[t]he muscles, so long dormant in my leg, begin to feel as if they reached the foot; the warm blood seems to again tingle in the toes, and the old sensations, long forgotten, again resume their sway'.[70] Another declared that it was 'so like the natural limb that we could look upon it with no feeling than that it was part and parcel of the human body'.[71] The term 'natural' was applied to the artificial leg, the amputated leg and the remaining leg alike, as the equation of form and function collapsed them together. In this formulation other modes of compensation beside the Palmer limb were surely less than natural, and perhaps less than human. With its mechanical and aesthetic ideals, its embodiment of American ingenuity and its capacity to restore men economically, socially and physically, the Palmer limb leveraged a nineteenth-century trust in all that technology and material consumption might do.

Conclusions

Palmer's publicity and advertising materials sketch the contours of a culture in which the artificial limb was a desirable consumer product, freighted with the promise of sociability, productivity and bodily wholeness. At its heart were the wearers themselves, whose testimonials, though probably heavily edited, constituted a kind of proto-community. Using the narrative form to make their bodies legible, many writers consciously directed their words to their fellow amputees. One wrote, for instance, '[I] cheerfully make this public declaration to the manufacturers, hoping it may meet the eye of some unfortunate brother, who will "go and do likewise"'.[72] Another concurred that '[m]isfortunes of our own naturally excite in us a sympathy for those who are like situated, and hence it is that I would use my influence to induce those who may have suffered the loss of a limb to procure one of "Palmer's Patent"'.[73] Artificial limb wearers created a community that used the social power of technology and consumption to speak back to their fears about dependency and isolation.

This community and its voice extended outward too, reaching exhibition visitors and readers of *Punch* and *The Times* with the promise of a commodity that could resolve the anxieties of bodily difference and the risk of an unproductive life. The consumer product was so desirable that, despite persistent injunctions to hide their missing limbs, wearers might actually choose to show off their replacements. Palmer's 'six gentlemen' figuratively demonstrated the quality and function of their appliances, their bodies and their manliness. Another testimonial boasted of the limb almost as a status symbol: '[e]very one to whom I have shown it, is delighted with it as a work of art, and for its beauty of finish'.[74] Another man claimed that '[i]n my travels I have met with many individuals wearing artificial legs, but think I have found none whom I could not easily distance on a half mile heat'.[75] Within the pages of Palmer's advertising grew a recognition of bodily difference that did not simply force people into normative social participation, but also celebrated the process and its accessories: the technology of disability would not always be hidden or sneered at, but also sometimes praised for its mechanical and commercial sophistication and its social good.

The Palmer leg seemingly allowed the wearer to move from a passive position to an active one. Like Palmer himself, he might choose to show or to hide his bodily difference for social gain – to carry out performances of surprising ability or cool confidence. But this apparent opportunity for normative masculinity and productive living left little room for non-compliance. Palmer's product, and the accompanying articles and awards, made no allowance for those who might have found the prosthesis uncomfortable, unaffordable or simply unwanted. The onus of inclusion lay firmly with the wearer, who had no choice but to consume his way to apparent self-reliance and respect. The promised personal and social mastery were evinced, in the first instance, by the very act of buying the leg. The shop was the site of rebirth, evidenced by 'the numbers that flock to the proprietor's office ... upon crutches, with dejected countenances, and return walking upright and smiling'.[76] The bourgeois act of shopping confirmed that one was back in the market economy, the antithesis of the begging cripple crouched on the street corner. Putting product above problem made bodily difference little more than another opportunity for inclusion in a consumer society, but it also made consumption the *only* opportunity for inclusion for those with missing limbs. For these men, social belonging was surely vital, but it came at a high price: as much as $150 for a Palmer leg, as well as the incalculable cost of adhering to a relentless ideal of independent masculinity.

Notes

1 He may have been named after Benjamin Franklin (1706–90), one of the Founding Fathers of the United States, who was also known as an inventor.

2 B. F. Palmer, 'Artificial Leg' (United States [US] Patent Number 4834, 4 November 1846).

3 L. Figg and J. Farrell-Beck, 'Amputation in the Civil War: physical and social dimensions', *Journal of the History of Medicine and Allied Sciences*, 48 (1993), 454–75, at 454. For Civil War prostheses, see, for example, F. M. Clarke, *War Stories: Suffering and Sacrifice in the Civil War North* (Chicago, IL: University of Chicago Press, 2011); G. Hasegawa, *Mending Broken Soldiers: The Union and Confederate Programs to Supply Artificial Limbs* (Carbondale, IL: Southern Illinois University Press, 2012); L. Herschbach, 'Prosthetic reconstructions: making the industry, re-making the body, modelling the nation', *History Workshop Journal*, 44 (1997), 22–57; B. C. Miller, *Empty Sleeves: Amputation in the Civil War South* (Athens, GA: University of Georgia Press, 2015); M. K. Nelson, *Ruin Nation: Destruction and the American Civil War* (Athens, GA: University of Georgia Press, 2012), especially pp. 160–227; J. O. Padilla, 'Army of "Cripples": Northern Civil War Amputees, Disability, and Manhood in Victorian America' (unpublished PhD thesis, University of Delaware, 2007); D. D. Yuan, 'Disfigurement and reconstruction in Oliver Wendell Holmes's "The human wheel, its spokes and felloes"', in D. T. Mitchell and S. L. Synder (eds), *The Body and Physical Difference: Discourses of Disability in the Humanities* (Ann Arbor, MI: University of Michigan Press, 1997), pp. 71–88.

4 Palmer & Co, 'Offices of Palmer's patent leg and mechanical surgery', *American Medical Gazette*, 8 (1857), 768. About 500 of these belonged to women. The role of women and artificial limbs has been explored by, for example, V. Warne, '"To invest a cripple with peculiar interest": artificial legs and upper-class amputees at mid-century', *Victorian Review*, 35:2 (2009), 83–100 and C. Lieffers, '"Two good limbs": women and prostheses in nineteenth-century America', unpublished paper presented at 'Gender, Bodies and Technology', Women's Studies Conference, Blacksburg, VA, United States, 2 May 2014.

5 S. F. Rose, *No Right to Be Idle: The Invention of Disability, 1840s–1930s* (Chapel Hill, NC: University of North Carolina Press, 2017). For a general review of changes in the American economy and labour market in this period, see, among many others, D. R. Meyer, *The Roots of American Industrialization* (Baltimore, MD: Johns Hopkins University Press, 2003); D. A. Hounshell, *From the American System to Mass Production, 1800–1932: The Development of Manufacturing Technology in the United States* (Baltimore, MD: Johns Hopkins University Press, 1984); and W. Licht, *Industrializing America: The Nineteenth Century* (Baltimore, MD: Johns Hopkins University Press, 1995).

6 For more reflection on the cultural significance of testimonials, see M. Schweitzer and M. Moskowitz (eds), *Testimonials in the American Marketplace: Emulation, Identity, Community* (London: Palgrave Macmillan, 2009).

7 See, for example, K. Ott, 'The sum of its parts: an introduction to modern histories of prosthetics', in K. Ott, D. Serlin, and S. Mihm (eds), *Artificial Parts, Practical Lives* (New York, NY: New York University Press, 2002), pp. 1–42, at pp. 8–10. For an early study of the differences between the medical and social models, see M. Oliver, *The Politics of Disablement* (London: Macmillan Education, 1990).

8 This figure is based on statistics from Massachusetts General Hospital. See M. S. Pernick, *A Calculus of Suffering: Pain, Professionalism, and Anesthesia in Nineteenth-Century America* (New York, NY: Columbia University Press, 1985), p. 219.

9 'B. Frank Palmer's Portrait', *The Scalpel*, 5 (1854), 448–9, at 448. There is some confusion as to when Palmer lost his leg. *The Scalpel* reported age eleven, while Charles F. Stansbury suggested 1837 (making Palmer about thirteen) in *Argument in Behalf of the Extension of the Patent of B. Frank Palmer, for An Improvement in Artificial Legs* (Baltimore, MD: Murphy and Co., 1860), p. 5. The marquess of Anglesey reportedly used a version of James Potts's leg (patented in Britain in 1800), which Potts's apprentice, William Selpho, brought to the United States when he immigrated in 1839 (G. E. Marks, *A Treatise on Artificial Limbs with Rubber Hands and Feet* (New York, NY: A. A. Marks, 1896), p. 16).

10 'B. Frank Palmer's Portrait', 448.

11 See B. F. Palmer, *Artificial Leg* (US Patent Number 6122, 20 February 1849); B. F. Palmer, *Artificial Leg* (US Patent Number 9200, 17 August 1852); O. W. Holmes, 'The human wheel, its spokes and felloes', *Atlantic Monthly*, 11 (1863), 575; B. F. Palmer, 'Palmer's Patent Leg', *Peninsular Journal of Medicine and the Collateral Sciences*, 4:5 (1856), advertisement, p. 3.

12 Winnipissiogee, 'New Hampshire', *New York Daily Times*, 4 August 1853, p. 2.

13 J. Church *et al.*, 'Palmer's artificial leg', *Boston Medical and Surgical Journal*, 41 (1849), 44–5, at 44.

14 A. M. Richardson, letter, 1855, in B. F. Palmer and E. D. Hudson (eds), *The Artificial Leg Reporter and Surgical Adjuvant* (New York, NY: Palmer and Co, 1857), p. 21 (emphasis in original).

15 P. Starr, *The Social Transformation of American Medicine* (New York, NY: Basic Books, 1982), p. 54.

16 This argument is more thoroughly expounded in C. Lieffers, 'Itinerant manipulators and public benefactors: artificial limb patents, medical professionalism, and the moral economy in antebellum America', in C. L. Jones (ed.), *Rethinking Modern Prostheses in Anglo-American Commodity Cultures, 1820–1939* (Manchester: Manchester University Press, 2017), pp. 137–57.

17 Palmer and Co, 'Palmer's Patent Leg', *The Water-Cure Journal*, 18 (1855), 141.

18 B. F. Palmer, 'Subsidiary art', in Palmer and Hudson (eds), *The Artificial Leg Reporter and Surgical Adjuvant*, pp. 8–10, at p. 9.

19 B. F. Palmer 'On artificial limbs', *"Palmer's Patent" Artificial Leg Reporter and Surgical Adjuvant*, 2:2 (1850), 5–6, at 5; Palmer, 'Subsidiary art', 9.

20 Palmer, 'Subsidiary art', 9; E. D. Hudson, 'Anagraphs of surgical pathology and surgery of the extremities', *Surgical Adjuvant and Reporter of Artificial Limbs*, 9 (1859), 7–16, at 15.

21 'Jurors of the World's Great Exhibition, London, 1851', in B. F. Palmer, *The Palmer Arms and Leg, Adopted for the U.S. Army and Navy* (Philadelphia, PA: American Artificial Limb Company, 1865), p. 14.

22 'Palmer and Co's Artificial Leg, Springfield, Massachusetts', *The Scalpel*, 5 (1852), 56–7, at 57.

23 T. Richards, *The Commodity Culture of Victorian England: Advertising and Spectacle, 1851–1914* (Stanford, CA: Stanford University Press, 1990), p. 39.

24 Palmer and Co, 'Palmer's Patent Leg Manufactories', in D. E. Hall (ed.), *A Condensed History of the Origination, Rise, Progress, and Completion of the 'Great Exhibition of the Industry of all Nations'* (New York, NY: Redfield, 1852), n.p.

25 'Palmer's legs', *Punch*, 21 (1851), 137.

26 'Artificial limbs', *New York Daily Times*, 26 March 1855, p. 1; 'The Great Exhibition', *The Times*, 19 September 1851, p. 4.

27 'B. Frank Palmer's Portrait', 449. See also B. F. Palmer, 'Palmer's artificial leg in London', *Boston Medical and Surgical Journal*, 45 (1851), 18–22, at 21. The marquess apparently requested a Palmer leg even before the Exhibition: *American Cabinet and Boston Athenaeum*, quoted in 'Expressions of the Press', *"Palmer's Patent" Artificial Leg Reporter and Surgical Adjuvant*, 2:2 (1850), 11–14, at 12.

28 The resulting anxiety is well documented in contemporary newspapers. See, for example, 'The London Exhibition', *The Daily Ohio Statesman*, 24 April 1851, p. 2. For further analysis, see M. Curti, 'America at the World's Fairs, 1851–1893', *American Historical Review*, 55 (1950), 833–56; M. Cunliffe, 'America at the Great Exhibition of 1851', *American Quarterly*, 3 (1951), 115–26.

29 B. F. Palmer, 'Palmer's Patent Leg in London', *Boston Medical and Surgical Journal*, 45 (1851), 258–62, at 261.

30 'The Great Exhibition', *The Times*, 19 September 1851, p. 4.

31 Stansbury, *Argument in Behalf*, p. 5.

32 Palmer, 'Subsidiary Art', 8 (emphasis in original). See also A. A. Ekirch, *The Idea of Progress in America, 1815–1860* (New York, NY: Columbia University Press, 1944), especially pp. 106–31.

33 N. White, letter, 1850, *"Palmer's Patent" Artificial Leg Reporter and Surgical Adjuvant*, 2:2 (1850), 17.

34 A. de Tocqueville, *Democracy in America*, new edn (London: Longmans, Green, and Co, 1889), vol. 2, p. 120.

35 B. F. P., 'Infringements – caution', *The Surgical Adjuvant and Reporter of Artificial Limbs*, 9 (1859), 20–23, at 20 (emphasis in original).

36 G. G. Foster, *New York in Slices* (New York, NY: W. F. Burgess, 1849), p. 8.

37 'Palmer's patent leg is far superior', *Association Medical Journal*, 4 (1856), 400.

38 'Artificial Limbs', *New York Daily Times*, 26 March 1855, p. 1.

39 'Palmer and Co's artificial leg, Springfield, Massachusetts', p. 57; W. Hamilton, 'Report on Mr. B. F. Palmer's artificial leg', *Journal of the Franklin Institute*, 3rd series 19 (1850), 60–1, at 60.

40 S. Mihm, '"A limb which shall be presentable in polite society": prosthetic technologies in the nineteenth century', in K. Ott, D. Serlin, and S. Mihm (eds), *Artificial Parts, Practical Lives* (New York, NY: New York University Press, 2002), pp. 282–99.

41 'B. Frank Palmer's Portrait', 448; B. F. P. 'Ascending Mount Washington in a Storm', in B. F. Palmer (ed)., *Steps* (Philadelphia: B. F. Palmer, c. 1874), p. 96.

42 A. A. L. M. Velpeau, *New Elements of Operative Surgery*, trans. P. S. Townsend, 4th edn, 3 vols (New York, NY: Samuel S. & W. Wood, 1856), II, 276; also quoted in Palmer and Hudson (eds), *The Artificial Leg Reporter and Surgical Adjuvant*, p. 2.

43 Hamilton, 'Report on Mr B. F. Palmer's artificial leg', 60.

44 See E. Goffman, *Stigma: Notes on the Management of Spoiled Identity* (Englewood Cliffs, NJ: Prentice-Hall, 1963).

45 O. S. Fowler, *Private Lectures on Perfect Men, Women and Children* (Sharon Station, New York, NY: Mrs. O. S. Fowler, 1883), p. 27.

46 Stansbury, *Argument in Behalf*, p. 11.

47 See Erin O'Connor, *Raw Material: Producing Pathology in Victorian Culture* (Durham, NC: Duke University Press, 2000), pp. 124–5.

48 M. Zakim, *Ready-made Democracy: A History of Men's Dress in the American Republic, 1760–1860* (Chicago, IL: University of Chicago Press, 2003), p. 102; R. L. Bushman, *The Refinement of America: Persons, Houses, Cities* (New York, NY: Knopf, 1992), p. 361.

49 A. Ayres, *The Mentor: A Little Book for the Guidance of Such Men and Boys as Would Appear to Advantage in the Society of Persons of the Better Sort* (1884; New York, NY: D Appleton and Company, 1902), pp. 59–60.

50 'Palmer's artificial limbs', *Boston Medical and Surgical Journal*, 46 (1852), 513–15, at 515. Sanford's initials are sometimes given as J. M.

51 'An interesting case in mechanical surgery', *The American Medical Gazette and Journal of Health*, 8 (1857), 719–20.

52 O'Connor, *Raw Material*; Herschbach, 'Prosthetic reconstructions', 45 (emphasis in original).

53 Stansbury, *Argument in Behalf*, p. 10.

54 *Ibid.*

55 J. C. Moss, letter, 1855, in Palmer and Hudson (eds), *The Artificial Leg Reporter and Surgical Adjuvant*, 12 (emphasis in original).

56 R. G. Thomson, *Extraordinary Bodies: Figuring Physical Disability in American Culture and Literature* (New York, NY: Columbia University Press, 1997), p. 46.

57 Palmer & Co, 'Palmer's Patent Leg Manufactories', n.p. (emphasis in original).

58 'Palmer's artificial limbs', *Boston Medical and Surgical Journal*, 514.

59 Quoted in Stansbury, *Argument in Behalf*, p. 13.

60 E. A. Staniels, letter, 1861, in Palmer and Hudson (eds), *The Artificial Leg Reporter and Surgical Adjuvant*, p. 15.

61 S. W. Mitchell, 'Phantom limbs', *Lippincott's Magazine of Popular Literature and Science*, 8 (1871), 563–9.

62 P. Hubbell, letter, 1858, *Surgical Adjuvant and Reporter of Artificial Limbs*, 9 (1859), 39 (emphasis in original).

63 Junius [Calvin Colton], 'Labor and Capital', *Junius Tracts*, 7 (New York, NY: Greeley and McElrath, 1844), 111 and 105 (emphasis in original).

64 'Palmer's artificial limbs', *Scientific American*, 14:25 (1859), 208.

65 See Rose, *No Right*.

66 E. Wright, letter, 1856, in Palmer and Hudson (eds), *The Artificial Leg Reporter and Surgical Adjuvant*, 12.

67 Stansbury, *Argument in Behalf*, pp. 10, 12.

68 'Palmer's artificial limbs', *Boston Medical and Surgical Journal*, 514.

69 *New York State Republican*, quoted in 'Expressions of the Press', *"Palmer's Patent" Artificial Leg Reporter and Surgical Adjuvant*, 2:2 (1850), 11–14, at13.

70 F. H. Furniss, letter, 1874, in Palmer (ed.), *Steps*, p. 5 (original in italics).

71 *Buffalo Republic*, quoted in 'Expressions of the Press', *"Palmer's Patent" Artificial Leg Reporter and Surgical Adjuvant*, 2:2(1850), 11–14, at 13.

72 White, *"Palmer's Patent" Artificial Leg Reporter and Surgical Adjuvant*, 2:2, 17.

73 W. Werden, letter, 1850, in *The Orthopedic, or Artificial Leg Reporter and Surgical Adjuvant*, 5 (1852), 14.

74 J. A. Farnsworth, letter, 1847, *"Palmer's Patent" Artificial Leg Reporter and Surgical Adjuvant*, 2:2 (1850), 15.

75 T. Child Jr, letter, 1847, *"Palmer's Patent" Artificial Leg Reporter and Surgical Adjuvant*, 2:2 (1850), 15.

76 *Mechanic's Reporter*, quoted in 'Expressions of the Press', *"Palmer's Patent" Artificial Leg Reporter and Surgical Adjuvant*, 2:2 (1850), 11–14, at 13.

Part III

LEGACIES

8

THE DISABLED CHILD IN AN INDUSTRIAL METROPOLIS: GLASGOW'S CHILDREN'S HOSPITAL, SCOTTISH CONVALESCENT HOMES 'IN THE COUNTRY' AND EAST PARK HOME FOR INFIRM CHILDREN

Iain Hutchison

In the early nineteenth century Scotland remained a mainly rural, agricultural country, but one that was witnessing nascent industrial expansion as mineral resources such as coal and iron ore were exploited and advantage was taken of natural harbours and estuaries, close to centres of population, to exploit these resources. Development of heavy industry and associated transportation networks rapidly resulted in the transformation of Scotland from a predominantly rural society to a heavily urbanised one, concentrated in a resource-rich axis that ran from Ayrshire in the south-west, through Lanarkshire, Glasgow, the Lothians and Fife to Dundee in the east.[1] By the dawn of the Victorian era, towns and cities were increasing in population, but often within constricted boundaries. Prosperity arising from industry and trade benefited those with capital to invest. However, any prosperity gained by people who had only their labour to offer was tenuous. Glasgow, as the centre for much of Scotland's industrial growth, did not enjoy a healthy environment due to overcrowding in often insanitary conditions.[2] Glasgow therefore presents a useful case study for the exploration of institutional responses to children with poor health and disabling conditions in the Victorian era, and for observing how some of these responses continued through the twentieth century.

In Scotland, institutional strategies for sensory-impaired children began in the late eighteenth century.[3] These were followed by similar responses for mentally impaired children in the mid-nineteenth century.[4] An institutional approach for physically impaired children arrived later than for other forms of impairment, while in Glasgow provision of a children's hospital to treat conditions such as rickets and various tubercular diseases was also a late innovation compared with other large European cities.[5] This chapter will focus on Glasgow's Royal Hospital for Sick Children, its use of a network of convalescent homes for frail and impaired children and its enduring links with East Park Home, an institution created to aid children with a range of disabling conditions. In tracing the development and interaction of these interventions, it will demonstrate Victorian responses to aiding the plight of the disabled child and show how these responses endured in the twentieth century.[6]

The battle for a children's hospital

By 1860, high infant mortality had become an all-too-readily accepted feature of Scottish industrial society. However, among Glasgow's medical profession there was growing concern about the large number of deaths among infants and children and the failure of the city to arrest the attrition arising from childhood diseases. As a consequence, a meeting was convened on 23 January 1861, attended by doctors and members of the city elite, to draw attention to the problem and propose a solution.

In particular, the gathering noted that 'the excessive rate of infantile mortality which prevails in Glasgow as shown by the reports of the Registrar General calls for the adoption of preventive measures'.[7] The preventive measure proposed by the gathering was that 'the most efficacious means of diminishing this mortality, [is] the institution of an hospital for the reception and treatment of sick children similar to those already established on the continent of Europe and in this country'.[8]

The first children's hospital, Hôpital des Enfants Malades, opened in Paris in 1802, and this was followed by the Institute for Sick Children, Dublin (1821), St Anna's Children's Hospital, Vienna (1837) and the Hospital for Sick Children, London (1852). In the United States, the Children's Hospital of Philadelphia opened in 1855, while in the Scottish capital, Edinburgh, a twenty-bed children's hospital opened in 1860, a landmark which particularly stirred the sensitivities of those assembled for the Glasgow meeting because of traditional rivalry between the two cities.[9]

While awareness of the value of the child and the unacceptable level of infant and child mortality had been a recent development, the value of philanthropic endeavour to aid the deserving needy was well established.[10] Charity was used to fund the likes of Scotland's deaf and blind institutions, Baldovan Asylum for mentally impaired children near Dundee and hospitals such as Glasgow Royal Infirmary, which opened in 1794.[11] However, the directors of Glasgow Royal Infirmary (GRI) perceived proposals for a children's hospital to be a threat, partly because it might be expected to attract child patients to which the GRI felt it had claim, but especially as competition for the philanthropic support upon which it depended. Indeed, public largesse in supporting such institutions was so critical to their ability to exist, function and thrive that it was natural that the GRI would react decisively to protect its inward flow of revenue, as well as to defend its monopoly as the city's infirmary. These were the initial reasons that stalled the aspiration for a children's hospital in Glasgow from being turned into a reality.

In 1870 the University of Glasgow moved from the High Street, where its roots lay in the former medieval city, to the city's west end and where the new Western Infirmary would play a key role in the instruction of the university's medical students. This was initially seen by the children's hospital committee as an opportunity to embark on a programme of mutually beneficial cooperation with the university, its medical school and the Western Infirmary. Negotiations became protracted over several years and, ultimately, it was not until December 1882 that Glasgow's Hospital for Sick Children was formally declared open in a converted town-house, not in the west end, but in the centrally located district of Garnethill where it accepted its first patients during the following month.[12]

On 8 January 1883, five-year-old John Shields became the hospital's first admission, received to undergo treatment for spinal curvature. This 'deformity' was soon to be recorded as having 'disappeared on suspension' and he was discharged 'improved' three weeks later.[13] Shields's treatment and recovery had reached a fairly rapid conclusion; in 1883, 260 patients – 156 medical and 104 surgical – were admitted and their average length of stay was forty-three days.[14] Conditions treated included abscess, bronchitis, joint disease, poliomyelitis, tuberculosis of the lungs, and rickets.[15] The death rate among the children admitted in 1883 was 7.6 per cent. Published mortality rates in the years immediately following created unrealistic expectations among subscribers to the RHSC, and a consequent need for the directors to ascribe blame to outside factors, such as the too-late admission of very ill children.[16]

The case notes for the early admissions reveal the general health of these children's families and their living conditions in Glasgow. They provide descriptions of severe overcrowding in dwellings, of widespread chronic ill health, of infant and child morbidity and mortality, and of premature adult death. Case notes of children admitted to the hospital in its first year present numerous vignettes that narrate medical interventions and paediatric patient experience. For example, two-year-old Georgina McCaeadie had 'been in ill health for 17 months since she was weaned', two spells of enteritis (inflammation of the small intestine) had occurred while she was in the care of a wet nurse and she was described upon admission as ill-nourished and 'in a very weak state'. She was discharged 'cured' after a stay of seventeen weeks.[17] In the home of Charles McBeth, a seven-year-old with rickets, there were two siblings 'with legs the same description'.[18]

The need for the hospital was particularly highlighted by the case of eight-year-old Daniel Murchie, admitted on 22 January 1883. When he was four years old, Murchie's back was observed to be bent, and when he was six years old, an abscess had been drained at Glasgow's Western Infirmary. At the new children's hospital he was diagnosed with hip joint disease. Four days after admission, he was operated on. His case notes graphically describe the procedure:

> Today Dr MacEwan [*sic*] cut down and removed the head of the femur with a chain saw … The limb was put up with extension (4lbs). The old sinuses being scraped with Rothman's sharp spoon, bone dusted with Ioxoform. Considered an unfavourable case.[19]

The surgeon was William Macewen (1848–1924), and, despite a poor prognosis, within a month Murchie was apparently looking healthy, getting 'fat' and had colour in his cheeks. By 2 April 1883 he was 'up walking with aid of a "Go Cart"' and was discharged after a four-month stay.

The case of Daniel Murchie, who had languished for four years without serious surgical intervention, demonstrates the desperate need that prevailed for the children's hospital to cater for the paediatric needs of a major city burdened with poor health and with sub-standard housing for its constantly increasing population. Most early children's hospitals had developed from out-patient dispensaries in order that the more serious cases presented could be adequately treated. In Glasgow, the reverse occurred, it being the capacity limitation of the hospital that prompted moves to build a separate children's 'Dispensary and Outpatients'.

The creation of the Sick Children's Dispensary demonstrated Victorian philanthropy at its buoyant best and also showcases the under-acknowledged role of women – the wives and daughters of the rising urban upper-middle class and of the rural gentry and aristocracy – in raising finances for charitable endeavour while their husbands and fathers took the weighty decisions in sombre boardrooms about how public largesse should be invested in ameliorating child ill health. The directors discussed establishing an out-patient facility late in 1884, but the decisive initiative was taken by the indomitable Duchess of Montrose when she enquired where a dispensary should be located in order to serve the greatest need, the form it should take, the area of ground required and the estimated cost.[20]

Several possible sites for a dispensary were quickly identified and, on 6 February 1885, land was purchased a short distance from the hospital.[21] Meanwhile, the duchess had presented the directors with a cheque for £10,000 from the proceeds of a Fancy Fair. This event had been an amazing effort involving various middle-class and aristocratic women under the stewardship of the duchess. Derek Dow has observed that bringing the dispensary to fruition progressed 'with a speed which is bewildering to the twentieth-century mind resigned to bureaucracy and planning impasses.'[22] As its opening day approached in 1888, James Christie, medical officer for the Hillhead burgh of Glasgow, extolled its facilities and design:

> The patients are to be admitted by a court or covered way, where perambulators may be left protected from the weather, and this leads to a vestibule where they are to be registered and then transferred to the waiting-room, which is a large and airy apartment.[23]

The dispensary was designed to receive a large number of patients daily, and, while the hospital catered for hundreds annually, the dispensary was able to treat tens of thousands. In the words of Regius Professor of Surgery at the University of Glasgow, Sir George Macleod (1828–92), '[the dispensary] will meet the requirements of many cases which are unfitted for admission into the wards [and] ailments which are as yet slight, but which, if not attended to, would soon become aggravated and confirmed, can be here seen and treated.'[24]

While the dispensary served a need for children who might not otherwise secure a place in the wards of the hospital, another problem was identified during the early years of the institution. Children who had been treated needed time to recover; too-early discharge to poor housing conditions and diet could result in their recovery being arrested and reversed. Indeed, some children who had been successfully recovering in hospital went into rapid decline upon discharge to unfavourable living conditions, and for some, death followed. By 1900, there were consistently about eighty children on a waiting list for hospital admission, while further children identified as needing hospital treatment were being turned away by the dispensary owing to a lack of available beds. In order to provide recovery under hospital supervision while relieving demand for cots in the city-centre facility, a partial solution came through a philanthropic gesture by Miss Margaret Montgomery Paterson to build a 'country branch' in memory of her parents. This was encouraged by Mrs J. L. Mackie of the hospital's Ladies Committee, who offered £1,000 towards the project. This facility was intended to receive 'those children who ... occupy beds at the Hospital and yet do not require much active treatment', and it was considered 'that the change to the country will be highly beneficial to the more lingering

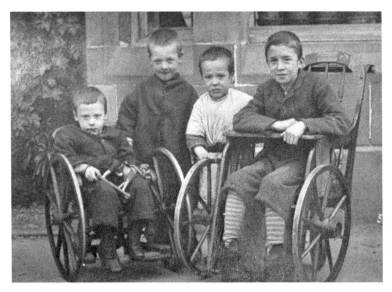

8.1 Children at the RHSC Country Branch. From the private collection of Elizabeth Anderson.

class of cases'.[25] In 1901 Miss Paterson committed £6,000 to the building of the Country Branch on a 1.5 acre site that had been identified close to the then-rural settlement of Drumchapel, a few miles west of the city. The Country Branch was to offer twenty-four beds in two wards and have accommodation for 'staff and servants'.[26] It opened in 1903, with Visiting Surgeon Robert Parry (1858–1943) commenting that 'the advantage to be gained by the treatment of many classes of cases in the fresh country air could not be over-estimated'.[27] The Country Branch was a direct extension of the hospital and increased the number of beds at its disposal by 25 per cent. Its erection and opening was achieved within a remarkably short time period and without the indecision and acrimony that had frustrated the original creation of the hospital and the founding of the dispensary.

The inauguration of the Country Branch provided relief, but not a solution, to high public demand for hospital cots. By the Edwardian period the hospital in Garnethill, close to Glasgow city centre, could no longer aspire to cope with the level of demand for its services. The directors embarked upon building a new, charitably funded, 200-bed hospital at Yorkhill, a former country estate overlooking the city's River Clyde with its docks and ship construction yards, but nonetheless considered to be in an airy, healthy environment. It opened in

1914 and within a decade was being proclaimed as 'The Biggest Children's Hospital in the Kingdom' and an institution that was making a major contribution to the scientific investigation of diseases affecting children, spreading knowledge as a teaching hospital, and training paediatric nurses – and, of course, providing direct medical and surgical treatment of infants and children.[28] Despite the onset of economic depression in the 1920s, the legacy of Victorian philanthropy remained active, through the likes of the RHSC, its Country Branch and its dispensary, until after the Second World War, in supporting children with ill health anrd disabling conditions.

Convalescent homes 'in the country'

The Country Branch of the RHSC was intended as a short-stay facility and it operated as a non-acute branch of the hospital. However, from the 1880s, the hospital also used convalescent homes to aid recovery through giving discharged children access to fresh air and a nourishing diet. This was especially critical for the many children who would otherwise return to impoverished families who lived in overcrowded city slums, many of which were single-room dwellings lacking sanitation, were pervaded by stale, polluted air and were deprived of natural light because of the close proximity of neighbouring tenements.[29]

The hospital's energetic Ladies Committee worked vigorously at fund-raising through its network of recruited volunteer lady collectors and made its presence felt in the hospital by visiting the children and overseeing the activities of the nursing staff. It was also the Ladies Committee that arranged convalescent facilities, for example in their conclusion of an arrangement with the Glasgow Poor Children's Fresh Air Fortnight organisation to send children 'to the country', usually in the neighbouring counties of Ayrshire, Buteshire, Dunbartonshire, Renfrewshire and Stirlingshire.[30] In 1891 the Ladies Committee arranged for 294 children to go 'to the country' from both the hospital and its outpatient dispensary, notably to Dundonald Home (108 children), Eaglesham (114), Fresh Air Fortnight Home (57), plus a small number to homes in Ayr, Helensburgh, Kilmun and Lenzie.[31]

The hospital had an arrangement with Glasgow's Trinity Congregational Church which began in 1890 when the church opened a convalescent home with ten cots at Eaglesham on the edge of Fenwick Moor, and initially under the care of Margaret Bartholomew, a former RHSC nurse.[32] In 1898 this home moved to a rural location between moor and sea above the port town of Greenock where it became known as Ravenscraig Children's Convalescent Home.[33] This was a ten-room 'cottage' run by Alice Buttercase, who had joined the hospital as a staff nurse in 1891, was promoted to Sister in 1894, and was described as an excellent worker when she left to become the home's matron in 1899.[34] In 1901 Buttercase was assisted by two domestic servants and the home housed thirteen children recovering from conditions including cardiac malfunction, cleft palate, hernia, pleurisy, chorea and amputation.[35]

RHSC patient records suggest that these children, nine of whom can be definitively traced in hospital ward ledgers, required a significant level of care at Ravenscraig Home. This is demonstrated by the case of Margaret Kane who moved back and forth between the hospital and Ravenscraig during her treatment for pelvic disease in 1900 and 1901. Her treatment culminated in amputation at the hip joint, followed by further convalescence at the home. Margaret's experience emphasises the disabling nature of some cases treated by the hospital, and also the role that this particular convalescent home played in providing an intermediate environment between hospital and return, in Margaret's case, to an overcrowded, two-room tenement dwelling occupied by nine people. Margaret Kane's childhood home circumstances were complex. She was born in 1893, but the 1891 census shows that six siblings had preceded her into the world, including a sister, Anne, who was recorded as being 'deaf and dumb'. A little over a year after Margaret's birth, her mother, listed as a widow, commenced a second marriage; Margaret's initial RHSC case note entry upon her admission on 9 January 1900, age six years and six months, declared her to be 'suffering from tubercular disease of left hip joint in early stage' and attributed her malady as arising after a fall twelve months earlier. Following Margaret's admission to the RHSC, numerous excisions to drain pus and scrape the bone were performed, but treatment culminated in amputation of her left leg at the hip joint in January 1901.[36]

These events were set against a background of impoverished living that had been further aggravated by the death of her father from consumption while she was an infant. The restructuring of family dynamics that followed could not have augured well for this child to survive and thrive and her impairment became increasingly serious. Yet, despite her poor prospects, it transpires that Margaret entered teenage employment as a dressmaker, married, had a family and lived until the grand age of ninety-one.[37]

Ravenscraig provided care for children who continued to require attentive nursing following discharge from the RHSC, and such convalescent homes reflected the philanthropic role played by churches, charities and sympathetically disposed individuals in supporting their existence. A formal agreement was drawn up between Ravenscraig and the RHSC in 1904 under which the home would accept children aged from two to twelve. This stated that the children should not require regular night attendance, had to be clean in person and clothing, be without infection or 'lung consumption', be able to get out of bed during the day and should not require more than superficial medical or surgical care.[38] This suggests that the home was becoming keen to avoid cases, such as Margaret Kane, with a potentially high level of care needed from staff. Under the agreement, the church paid all the expenses of the children and it was permitted to recommend admissions, but medical need was the final arbiter.[39] The hospital had almost exclusive access while being responsible for neither the running costs nor the day-to-day management of the home. This contrasted with other hospitals that managed their own convalescent homes, for example the Schaw Convalescent Home, which was bequeathed to Glasgow Royal Infirmary in 1898 following its construction by Miss Marjory Schaw (d. 1915) in memory of her brother, eminent Glasgow merchant Archibald S. Schaw (1819–89).[40]

Victorian philanthropy, often motivated by religiously inspired beliefs in the virtues of charitable acts, continued through the Edwardian era and it was the hard economic conditions of inter-war depression rather than a decline in compassion that saw Ravenscraig further restrict its admission policy in 1922. It now made the lower age limit four years and listed a range of medical conditions for which it did not wish to accept responsibility.[41] Medical conditions to be excluded from admission were: any infectious disease; active tuberculosis of the lung; progressive tuberculosis peritonitis; cardiac disease; unhealed empyema; faecal fistula; cerebral or meningeal conditions; infectious skin conditions; septic diseases of the bones, joints or cellular tissues; any of the incurable complications of tuberculous disease; and active tuberculosis of the bones, joints, skin or cellular tissues. However, in a more positive vein, it added that 'chronic forms of tuberculosis (e.g. of glands) even with limited discharge; or residual sinuses connected with healing tuberculous lesions or bones or of joints are to be regarded as in many cases eminently suitable for admission to and treatment in the Home'.[42]

The home was a facility of modest size and limited resources, and Ravenscraig's management committee was anxious that, aside from concern about control of infection, the children it received did 'not require medical or surgical treatment saving simple medicines and dressings,' this of course being in harmony with its objective of providing post-treatment convalescence in a healing environment.[43] In 1926 the home found itself in financial difficulties and under threat of closure. This was averted by the RHSC now undertaking to pay a subscription of five shillings weekly for each child.[44] The relationship between the hospital and Ravenscraig Home therefore became increasingly intertwined. The value of Ravenscraig was reaffirmed in 1939 when the RHSC almoner, who was employed by the hospital but appointed by the Ladies Committee, recorded that immediate vacancies could often be arranged 'for a child leaving the wards who would otherwise have to return to home conditions unsuitable for a patient just out of hospital'.[45]

With the onset of the Second World War, several convalescent homes, most notably Ravenscraig, were unable to continue operating due to funding crises or war-time requisition of their property for alternative use.[46] While there are deficiencies in the recording of statistics for children placed by the RHSC in convalescent homes, it would appear that such placements reached a peak in 1933 with 355 admissions, of which 167 were to Ravenscraig.[47]

While convalescent homes had become increasingly cautious in their admission policies because of perceived, and genuine, limitations in their abilities to cope with children with complex medical needs, one institution that catered for children requiring intensive nursing for conditions such as pulmonary tuberculosis and rickets was the Children's Home Hospital in Stirlingshire.[48] This had its beginnings in Aberfoyle in 1903 when the aura of the recently deceased Queen Victoria was high in the national consciousness, but in 1913 it relocated to Strathblane.[49] The founding aim of the Children's Home Hospital was to help 'make useful citizens of those whose lives would otherwise be a source of misery and weariness to themselves and their guardians'.[50] An example of a child patient transferred from the RHSC to Strathblane was cited by almoner Margaret Watson in 1929:

> M.N. was a nervous child who had attended the Hospital since she was four years old with symptoms of St Vitus Dance. Her mother had died of meningitis, and her father was in the Navy, and M.N. was looked after by her grandmother … Her heart was beginning to show signs of strain, and it was felt that she must be removed from her home surroundings. The first available vacancy in the rheumatism ward at Strathblane was secured for her, and she is now reported to be making progress there.[51]

The Strathblane facility had a longer-term caring role than the RHSC Country Branch, and gave a more intensive level of medical care than typical 'convalescence' while displaying many of the features of homes such as Ravenscraig. It was fully absorbed into the RHSC upon the creation of the state-funded National Health Service from 1948, and in the latter decades of the twentieth century the Children's Home Hospital provided long-term care for children and adolescents with conditions ranging from rickets to spina bifida. In 1994 changes in government strategy saw its closure and its young adults were moved to supported independent-living accommodation 'in the community'. This Edwardian institution, which had been founded on the enduring Victorian ethos of religiously inspired charity, and with aims of endowing its children with the capacity for 'self-help', had played an evolving role that

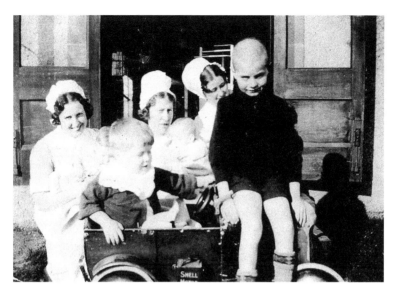

8.2 East Park Home boys, late 1880s. From the private collection
of Iain Hutchison.

sustained it four years beyond the end of Margaret Thatcher's 'Victorian values'
premiership.[52]

East Park Home for Infirm Children

During 1947, the RHSC's final year as a charitable institution, 210 children
were placed in convalescent homes, of which the largest number, 53, were
received by the specialist East Park Home for Infirm Children in Maryhill,
Glasgow and its country branch in Largs, Ayrshire.[53] By this time a relationship between RHSC and East Park Home had become well established. In its
1929 annual report East Park Home's physician superintendent, A. Bankier
Sloan, wrote:

> The Royal Hospital for Sick Children is making more and more use of the Home
> for cases requiring prolonged convalescent care, and in doing so, testifies to the
> useful function the Home fulfils. Fully 50 patients were received from Yorkhill
> [the hospital] and West Graham Street [the dispensary] last year [1929]. Quite
> a large proportion of these cases were heart cases, and in receiving them we are
> a unit in the campaign at present being waged against the dire effects of rheumatism
> in childhood.[54]

East Park Home was opened in 1874 to provide care for disabled children found living, often in squalid conditions, without the medical or nutritional aid that they badly needed.[55] Awareness of many of these children had been generated by the 1872 Education (Scotland) Act, which required compulsory education of all children aged between five and thirteen, and the consequential role of attendance officers in seeking out children who were failing to attend school. The founding organisation, the Association for Visiting and Aiding Permanently Infirm and Imbecile Children, quickly discovered that caring intervention within domestic dwelling places was inadequate for some of the children encountered. Echoing a point made in this volume by Martin Atherton (Chapter 10), the Association was forthright in pontificating about families whom it considered deserving and non-deserving, declaring that the parents of many of these children were 'intemperate, thoughtless, and very indifferent to the[ir] sad condition.'[56]

On 17 August 1874 the Association's directors discussed a proposal to purchase a 'cottage' 'suitable for the accommodation of about fifty children' – a plan that was quickly fulfilled so that, by 9 October, alterations and adaptions had been undertaken, staff had been employed and the first eleven children had been admitted to the newly acquired 'cottage'.[57] Yet, East Park Home was intended only 'as a temporary Institution … until such times as the Cottage Homes are ready, which it is proposed to erect in the National Institution being proposed by Miss Clugston' – a reference to the efforts of one of its committee members, philanthropist Beatrice Clugston (1827–88), and which came to fruition with the opening of the Broomhill Home for Incurables at Kirkintilloch in 1876.[58] Initially, East Park Home received children with sensory and mental impairments, alongside those with physical impairments, although this policy was adapted upon the early realisation that it made sense to direct appropriate children to existing deaf institutions, blind asylums, Baldovan Institution for Treatment and Education of Imbecile Children and the Scottish National Institution for the Education of Imbecile Children, at Larbert, Stirlingshire.[59]

Scope for East Park Home and the RHSC to work together was particularly realised when a department for making splints and other medical and surgical appliances was opened at the hospital in 1919.[60] East Park Home found benefits in being able to refer its children to the hospital for orthopaedic appliances, while, from around 1927, RHSC increasingly valued the specialist nature of East Park Home as a recipient of child patients with disabling conditions who needed long-term residential and educational support, and which was to increasingly include children with conditions such as chronic rheumatism and heart disease.[61] However, there was not always a harmonious relationship between East Park Home and the RHSC. The East Park Home directors sensed that the hospital was interested in receiving only 'curable' cases, leaving the home to aid seriously disabled children 'not received by the Sick Children's Hospital' as best they could manage.[62] This perception by the East Park Home directors resonates with the observations made by Amy Farnbach Pearson (see Chapter 1) on the objectives of Scottish adult voluntary hospitals.

Of course, it served a charitable body such as East Park Home well in its fund-raising efforts if the directors could plead that it was alone and unique in addressing an area of deserving and neglected need. However, benefactors of one institution were often found to be supporting others. When it came to large philanthropic efforts, we find that the Duchess of Montrose, who had driven the herculean fund-raising effort to bring about the Dispensary and Outpatients Department for the RHSC in the 1880s, was in action at East Park Home in 1896 with another grand fund-raising bazaar 'for the purpose of raising £3,000'.[63] At this point, the home had eighty-three children resident, presenting a significant range of impairing conditions and including spine disease (23 cases), paralysis (19), hip-joint disease (12), general struma (10) and rickets (16).[64]

In 1910 East Park Home explored the possibility of raising funds to create a country branch of its own, while, simultaneously, the convalescent home in Aberfoyle was seeking a new site to which it could relocate. In a typescript attachment to the 1910 annual report for East Park Home, its secretary, William Bunting, proposed negotiations to absorb the Aberfoyle Home Hospital, 'as the objectives of the Institutions are practically identical'.[65] Tellingly, Bunting also wrote of the Aberfoyle Home Hospital that he thought 'it might be unfortunate were there to be created a permanent institution of this kind, were its work to overlap with East Park' – thus the East Park Home overture was, in effect, an attempted hostile takeover.[66]

The aspiration by East Park Home for monopoly, not just in service provision to physically impaired children but as the primary or sole recipient of charitable giving for this category of child, had certain echoes of GRI's self-interest five decades earlier, when, in 1861, the idea of a children's hospital had first been mooted – and had been opposed by the GRI directors. However, absorption of Aberfoyle Home Hospital by East Park Home was repelled and, as mentioned earlier, the Aberfoyle Home Hospital relocated from Aberfoyle to Strathblane in 1913, and was integrated into the RHSC in 1948.

One RHSC patient from East Park Home during the inter-war period was Amy.[67] In oral testimony Amy described several visits from the home to the splints department at the RHSC.[68] Various procedures were undertaken to stimulate her mobility, which had been impaired by infantile paralysis, and included both the construction of orthopaedic boots and surgical intervention. As a child, Amy was early to develop awareness of her own agency and she became adept at speaking up for her rights and being perceptive of decisions affecting her well-being. She averred that surgical intervention was not a great success and said that a surgeon had confided that unsuccessful early procedures precluded her from benefiting from later developments because of damage done to ligaments during previous treatment. She was particularly upset that her father had not been consulted in order to give his permission for surgery, and her testimony highlights the way in which parents were expected to defer to health experts' and philanthropic guardians' knowledge, wisdom and good intentions. William Morton Fyfe, who was a medical student at RHSC in 1944 and returned as a registrar after qualification, acknowledged this patient and parental deference to clinicians: 'I felt that the parents trusted you entirely. Now whether that was fully justified or not is another matter, but I think they trusted you entirely and they were grateful for what you did for them.'[69] Amy was therefore, arguably, a victim of lay deference to the prevailing clinical monopoly of decision making in medical matters.

In 1927, when East Park's medical superintendent commented on continuing cooperation with the RHSC 'in receiving cases requiring prolonged care', the home in Maryhill, through years of development and expansion, had seen the original 'cottage' dwarfed by the addition of large adjoining villas, and in that year a country branch opened in the Ayrshire coastal town of Largs where sixty to seventy children could receive recuperative care at any one time.[70] Despite the gradual expansion of public health authorities, East Park Home, like the RHSC, was sustained by charitable giving where wealthy philanthropists enjoyed the privilege of dispensing largesse as entrenched in the Victorian spirit, and affluent middle-class localities were targeted for annual subscriptions by lady collectors. While East Park Home could not stand accused of openly engaging in Christian evangelism in the prosecution of its work, as the matrons' reports indicate, it is apparent that the support role, both financial and altruistic, continued to benefit considerably from churches, Sunday schools, mission schools and other religiously motivated groups.[71]

In the aftermath of the Second World War, East Park Home, like the RHSC, entered new eras. Today, a century and a half after East Park Home opened as a 'temporary' residential institution for children with severe disabling conditions, it continues as East Park School, providing education, occupational training and other forms of support for young people with impairments. It will be remembered that it was the introduction of compulsory education in 1872 that prompted East Park's founding. Victorian values were at the core of what its founders sought to achieve and this ethos had considerable longevity as the home's guiding ethos. But, inevitably, East Park has had to adapt over the decades and the disabling conditions for which it caters have changed. Instead of rickets, or tuberculosis of the bones, East Park's children now present with such conditions as cerebral palsy, and benevolently intended institutional intervention has given way to support for independent living for its young people and recognition of their rights to make their own choices and decisions.

Conclusion

Ravenscraig Convalescent Home, and many similar charitably funded rural retreats for post-operative recovery, had closed by the time of the creation of the National Health Service in 1948, a process that had been hastened to some degree by both the economic depression of the 1920s and 1930s and by widespread Second World War requisition of medical and residential property for military use. East Park Home, however, continued to be an important refuge for children with disabling conditions, and indeed the links between East Park and the hospital were further strengthened in 1951 when RHSC physician Robert Shanks took on the additional role of physician-superintendent to the home.[72] In the twenty-first century, children and young people continue to attend East Park School, while being provided with supported independent living in the local community.

The RHSC, East Park Home for Infirm Children, and a network of children's convalescent homes evolved to serve Glasgow and its industrial hinterland during the latter decades of the nineteenth century. The boundaries between illness and disability were often blurred, but it is apparent that children who entered the hospital as ill or infirm often endured long-term or permanently disabling conditions. Because of home conditions unfavourable to their post-treatment recovery, they were sent to a variety of intermediate places that provided a regime of fresh air and good diet. These included short-term convalescent homes that, despite preferring children whose medical circumstances would make them easy to care for, did accept children, such as Margaret Kane, who had severe disabling conditions. They included the RHSC's own Country Branch for short-term recuperation and, from 1948, the Children's Home Hospital for children and young adults requiring a place of residential support that might become their home for several years. From the inter-war period, a close relationship developed between the RHSC and East Park Home for Infirm Children where residential and education support was provided for children with a broad and changing spectrum of impairing conditions, and which continues today as an educational facility for children with disabilities while also supporting their independent living arrangements.

All of these facilities were founded in the Victorian era with the support of networks of people from the comfortable classes, many of whom were inspired in their support by religious conviction as well as by concern for defenceless and innocent children whose misfortunes in being impaired were aggravated by circumstances of poverty. The resilience of charitable giving came under pressure in the twentieth century because of economic depression and two world wars. Subsequently, the need for charity might have been expected to be challenged by the creation of a National Health Service in 1948, but those at the centre of charitable organisations found new roles that they might play, and they continued their philanthropic intervention in the Victorian tradition, particularly in such spheres as supporting disabled children. It was not until late in the twentieth century that the roles of 'Victorian' philanthropy were increasingly usurped by professional fund-raising bodies, but still marshalling the ethos and sentiment of Victorian charitable giving in their twenty-first-century rhetoric.

Notes

1 T. M. Devine, C. H. Lee and G. C. Peden (eds), *The Transformation of Scotland: The Economy since 1700* (Edinburgh: Edinburgh University Press, 2005).

2 A. K. Chalmers, *The Health of Glasgow, 1818–1925* (Glasgow: Corporation of Glasgow 1930); I. Maver, *Glasgow* (Edinburgh: Edinburgh University Press, 2000).

3 I. Hutchison, *A History of Disability in Nineteenth-century Scotland* (Lewiston: Edwin Mellen Press 2007); I. Hutchison, 'Oralism – a sign of the times? The contest for deaf communication in late nineteenth century Scotland', *European History Review*, 14:4 (2007); G. Phillips, *The Blind in British Society: Charity, State and Community, c. 1780–1930* (Aldershot: Ashgate, 2004).

4 I. Hutchison, 'Institutionalization of mentally-impaired children in Scotland, 1855–1914', *History of Psychiatry*, 22:4 (2011), 416–33.

5 I. Hutchison, 'Voices from the past: early institutional experience of children with disabilities – the case of Scotland', *Pediatric Rehabilitation*, 8.1 (January–March 2005), 66–77.

6 See also I. Hutchison, M. Nicolson and L. Weaver, *Child Health in Scotland: A History of Glasgow's Royal Hospital for Sick Children* (Erskine: Scottish History Press, 2016).

7 Greater Glasgow & Clyde Health Board Archives (hereafter GGCHBA), YH1/2/1, Royal Hospital for Sick Children (hereafter RHSC) Minutes of Board of Management 1861–1884, p. 2.

8 *Ibid.*, pp. 2–3.

9 Comparisons of child mortality figures between and within the two cities do not allow for differences in housing conditions, population density, poor sanitation, poverty, air pollution and numerous other variables. In January 1861, Glasgow, population 395,503, recorded 619 deaths of children under the age of five; Edinburgh, population 170,444, recorded 150 deaths. In January 1871, the comparative figures were Glasgow, population 491,846 – 678 deaths; and Edinburgh, population 196,991 – 168 deaths.

For the whole of 1881, Glasgow, population 511,415, recorded 5,365 child deaths under five years, while Edinburgh, population 228,373, recorded 1,688 deaths. Death rates were highest during the first two years of life, an age group which the paediatric hospitals did not normally receive. During the nineteenth century, neither city's paediatric hospital made claims of being able to make a noticeable impact on child mortality rates within its respective catchment area. *Monthly Returns of the Births, Deaths, and Marriages registered in the eight principal towns of Scotland ...* (HMSO), Jan 1861, p. 3, and Jan 1871, p. 3; *Twenty-seventh detailed annual report of the Register General of Births, Deaths, and Marriages in Scotland [Abstracts of 1881]* (HMSO, 1884), p. 30.

10 O. Checkland, *Philanthropy in Victorian Scotland* (Edinburgh: John Donald, 1980).

11 J. Jenkinson, M. Moss and I. Russell, *The Royal: The History of the Glasgow Royal Infirmary, 1794–1994* (Glasgow: Bicentenary Committee of Glasgow Royal Infirmary, 1994).

12 Hutchison *et al.*, *Child Health in Scotland*, pp. 26–40.

13 GGCHBA, YH7/2/1, RHSC Ward Journal, Case No. 1.

14 GGCHBA, YH3/1/1, RHSC Annual Report, 1883, p. 19.

15 *Ibid.*, pp. 20–1.

16 *Ibid.*, p. 19.

17 GGCHBA, YH7/4/1, RHSC Ward Journal, Case No. 31.

18 GGCHBA, YH7/2/1, RHSC Ward Journal, Case No. 26.

19 *Ibid.*, Case No. 20.

20 GGCHBA, YH1/2/2, RHSC Minutes of Board of Management 1884–1896, 26 December 1884, pp. 30–1.

21 GGCHBA, YH1/2/2, RHSC Minutes of Board of Management 1884–1896, 6 February 1885, pp. 43–4.

22 D. A. Dow, *The Dispensary of the Royal Hospital for Sick Children Glasgow* (Glasgow: Department of Clinical Physics and Bio-Engineering, 1980), p. 2.

23 J. Christie, *The Medical Institutions of Glasgow* (Glasgow: Maclehose, 1888), p. 69.

24 GGCHBA, YH3/1/1, RHSC Report of the Proceedings of the Opening of the Dispensary, Reports 1883–1891, p. 7.

25 GGCHBA, YH3/1/3, RHSC Annual Report y/e 31 December 1900, pp. 9–10.

26 GGCHBA, YH3/1/3, RHSC Annual Report y/e 31 December 1901, p. 10.

27 GGCHBA, YH3/1/3, RHSC Annual Report y/e 31 December 1903, p. 10.

28 *The Nursing Times*, 24 May 1924.

29 See P. Fyfe, *Back Lands and Their Inhabitants* (Glasgow, 1901), and Chalmers, *The Health of Glasgow*.

30 GGCHBA, YH1/2/2, 'RHSC Minutes of Board of Management 1884–1896', 11 June 1889, p. 188.

31 GGCHBA, YH3/1/1, RHSC Ninth Annual Report RHSC 1891, p. 11. For a comprehensive survey of convalescence homes, see J. Cronin, 'The Origins and Development of Scottish Convalescent Homes, 1860–1939' (PhD thesis, University of Glasgow, 2003).

32 GGCHBA, YH3/1/1, RHSC Annual Report 1890, p. 9; GGCHBA, YH8/1/1, Nurses Register.

33 GGCHBA, YH3/1/2, RHSC Annual Report 1898, p. 12. In 1898, eighty children passed through Ravenscraig Home from the Hospital and a further nine from the Dispensary.

34 GGCHBA, YH8/1/1, RHSC Register of Nurses and Students 1882–1902.

35 1901 Census, Civil Parish of Inverkip, Renfrewshire.

36 GGCHBA, YH7/3/11, RHSC Ward Journals – Medical Ward 3, pp. 97–8 and YH7/3/12, RHSC Ward Journals – Medical Ward 3, pp. 58–9, 135.

37 The reconstruction of Margaret Kane's life has been aided by examination of birth, marriage and death records and enumerators' books for the decennial censuses.

38 GGCHBA, RHSC Minute Book No. 4, 14 March 1905, pp. 105–11.

39 *Ibid.*

40 GGCHBA, HB14/2/10, Glasgow Royal Infirmary Annual Report, 1898, p. 8. A critique of Schaw Convalescent Home is given by J. Cronin in 'The Schaw Convalescent Home at Bearsden: not another costly pile', *Scottish Archives*, 23 (2017), 48–65. Neither Marjory Schaw nor her brother, Archibald Schaw, married. They lived in an opulent, four-storey terraced dwelling, with in excess of twenty rooms, at 26 Park Gardens, Glasgow, and were attended by three or four servants. Their living circumstances provide a stark contrast with those of the working-class poor in late-Victorian Glasgow, Source: decennial census returns, 1871–91.

41 GGCHBA, YH3/1/7, RHSC Memorandum and Articles of Association of The Royal Hospital for Sick Children, Incorporated 1st February 1922, p. 161, Memorandum of Agreement between the Directors of the Royal Hospital for Sick Children, Glasgow, and the Committee of Management of Trinity Church Convalescent Home for Children at Ravenscraig, Renfrewshire.

42 *Ibid.,* p. 162.

43 *Ibid.*

44 GGCHBA, RHSC Minute Book No. 9, 8 Nov 1926, p. 111; 8 Aug 1927, p. 180.

45 GGCHBA, YH3/1/11, RHSC Annual Report 1939, p. 37.

46 *Ibid.* In 1939, four unnamed convalescent homes were no longer able to receive children. Ravenscraig received 147 children from RHSC in 1940.

47 GGCHBA, YH3/1/10, RHSC Annual Report 1933, p. 41.

48 The Children's Home Hospital, originally an independent charitable institution, was acquired by the RHSC upon the creation of the National Health Service in 1948.

49 GGCHBA, HB12/2/14, The Children's Home Hospital Strathblane (late Aberfoyle), pp. 1, 3–5.

50 *Ibid.,* p. 6.

51 GGCHBA, YH3/1/9, RHSC Annual Report 1929, p. 36.

52 For the classic mid-Victorian 'liberal' doctrine of self-help, see S. Smiles, *Self-Help* (1859).

53 GGCHBA, YH3/1/12, RHSC Annual Report 1947, p. 20.

54 East Park School (hereafter EPS), East Park Home for Infirm Children (hereafter EPH) 56th Annual Report, Jan 1930, p. 7.

55 For an overview see P. Simpson, 'East Park Home for Infirm Children, Maryhill, Glasgow, 1874–1985', unpublished Diploma in Special Needs dissertation, Jordanhill College of Education (Feb 1985).

56 EPS, Association for Visiting and Aiding Permanently Infirm and Imbecile Children (hereafter AVAPIIC), Statement of the Object and Purpose of the Association (1874).

57 EPS, AVAPIIC Minute Book 1, 17 Aug and 9 Oct 1874.

58 *Ibid.*, 7 April 1874.

59 *Ibid.*, 6 Nov 1874.

60 GGCHBA, YH3/1/7, RHSC Annual Report 1919, p. 18.

61 EPS, EPH 56th Annual Report, Jan 1930, p. 7; GGCHBA, RHSC Annual Reports, 1914–1947.

62 EPS, EPH 35th Annual Report, Oct 1909, p. 5.

63 EPS, EPH 21st Annual Report, Oct 1895, pp. 3–4 and back cover.

64 *Ibid.*, p. 3.

65 EPS, EPH 36th Annual Report, Sep 1910, typescript attachment, p. 2.

66 *Ibid.*, p. 1.

67 Not her real name.

68 See, for example, Hutchison, 'Voices from the past'.

69 RHSC oral history interview with William Morton Fyfe (b. 1923), 5 Sep 2011.

70 EPS, EPH 54th Annual Report, Jan 1928, pp. 4, 8–9.

71 *Ibid.*, p. 12.

72 EPS, EPH 81st Annual Report, Jan 1952, pp. 8–10.

9

THE PANOPTICON: TOWARDS AN INTIMATE HISTORY OF SPECIAL SCHOOLS FOR THE BLIND

Fred Reid

The title of this chapter points to a significant gap in the historiography of residential special schools for the blind in Britain.[1] As it stands, the literature throws much light on this history: establishment of the schools around Britain; patterns of recruitment of students, as between for example 'blind' and 'partially sighted'; curriculum development and delivery; methods of teaching blind children, including the teaching of braille. The gap to which I wish to draw particular attention concerns sexual relationships between adolescent students in coeducational schools, many of whom spent most of their early years growing up in them.

The historiography has little to say on this topic. A partial exception is Sally French's oral history of the education of visually impaired people.[2] Her book contains sixty-one interviews with students, most of whom were educated in residential special schools before, during and after the Second World War. Some of these remark on the lack of sex education in their schools, the repressive rules and the adverse effect all this had on their subsequent lives. Understandably, these observations are brief and go little beyond matters of fact. On the whole they confirm the key aspects of my own experience: absence of formal sex education, repression of sexual relationships and severe punishment of transgression. Inevitably, however, the testimonies do not reflect on the reasons for such a regime and French has nothing to say on such questions.

I wrote my novella, *The Panopticon*, to fill this gap. It reflects the experience of my wife and myself when we were students in the Royal Blind School, Edinburgh, from 1952 to 1959.[3] In this chapter I explore three major themes arising from the novella. Firstly, I offer some biographical information to indicate the points of similarity and difference between our life stories and that of the two main characters of the fiction. Secondly, I discuss the origination of *The*

Panopticon, which grew out of the post-graduate MA course I taught on Historical Discourse and Methods at the University of Warwick. In this course we were reflecting on Michel Foucault's theory of the asylum. I then criticise Foucault's theory for ignoring the enhancement of life chances that the Royal Blind School afforded to many of its students in the period under review. Thirdly, I turn to the topic of sexual relationships, where I believe Foucault's theory of the carceral institution has some explanatory power, although even here with important qualifications. This leads me finally to some brief remarks on the relevance of my novella as a heuristic tool for historical writing on this topic in the history of special education.

I was born in 1937 and went blind following double detachment of the retina at the age of fourteen, going on fifteen, in 1952. In September of that year I became a pupil at the Royal Blind School (RBS), Edinburgh, familiarly known as 'Craigmillar' because of its location on the main road running to that district. The school was residential and coeducational, with a roll of about 120 children between ages two and eighteen. Some of us were totally blind – 'totals', we called each other – but perhaps about half were partially sighted, ranging from very low residual vision 'partials' to print-reading ability 'good partials'.

Boys and girls were rigidly segregated between floors for dormitories and at separate tables for meals in the dining hall. However, we were taught in mixed-sex classes, streamed by ability and designated, according to the educational classification of those days, 'senior' and 'junior' secondary. My senior secondary class was about twelve in number, pupils around my own age, about six of each sex. Senior secondary pupils were understood to be on a professional or commercial track. Junior secondary was loosely thought of as leading to industrial employment, still mostly in sheltered workshops. I soon fell in love with a girl of my own age, a student in my class. Etta had been blinded by a street accident at age six, and entered Craigmillar a year later. She stood out for me among the girls by her high spirits and lively curiosity. Our relationship lasted until we left Craigmillar at the age of twenty, Etta to train as a physiotherapist in London and I to study history at the University of Edinburgh. It survived this separation and we married in 1964. We had three sighted children within fifteen months, first a boy, then twin girls. I taught history for thirty-one years at the University of Warwick and Etta worked as a physiotherapist in Oxford, London and Leamington Spa. We both retired in 1997.

The birth of *The Panopticon*

I began to contemplate telling the intimate history of our lives at Craigmillar while teaching a talented group of post-graduate students in the mid-1990s.

We were reading together the works of Michel Foucault (1926–84). We discussed his theories of 'power-knowledge', of the 'carceral institution', of the 'archaeological' method of historical enquiry, of the modern 'episteme' and of 'the underground resistances' it provoked.[4] My students were very sympathetic to these theses, I less so. I began to realise that I had had experience of a carceral institution myself. Craigmillar had been a 'panopticon', the name philosopher Jeremy Bentham (1748–1832) gave to his design for 'an inspection house' which, he said, was 'applicable to any sort of establishment, in which persons of any description are to be kept under inspection; and in particular to penitentiary-houses, prisons, poor-houses, lazarettos, houses of industry, manufactories, hospitals, work-houses, mad houses, and schools'.[5] Foucault famously took up this idea as a model of the carceral institution as he understood it.

I recalled that, in the 1970s, we campaigners for inclusive education had likened special schools for the blind to 'prisons'. It now seemed to me that Foucault's theories went some way to accounting for the phenomenon. RBS certainly tried hard to control our bodies, more particularly our sexuality, by a regime of surveillance. As in Bentham's panopticon, the guards could always see the prisoners and they (at least the totals) could not see the guards. Many seemed, on that account, to internalise the rules of the school, which strictly forbade the slightest physical contact between the pupils on pain of expulsion as the ultimate penalty. On the other hand, there was, to use a Foucauldian term, a significant underground resistance among the pupils, some of whom joyfully engaged in clandestine sexual activity. It took the form, in our case (and, I believe, most others) of the restrained practices described by Szreter and Fisher in *Sex before the Sexual Revolution*.[6]

This idea grew in my mind until I sat down in about 1994 and wrote *The Panopticon*. Why did I choose a fictional rather than autobiographical form? In the first place, I wanted to give a truthful representation of a special school at that time without causing embarrassment by naming anyone. For that purpose, I adopted, in the first nine chapters of the novella, a highly naturalistic style. My school contemporaries who have read it comment on the vivid realisation of the setting and characters. Accordingly, *The Panopticon* has at least this historical value: it documents much that actually happened at Craigmillar – the indoor and outdoor games, such as football and cricket, the formal dances, the segregated accommodation in dormitories and, after sixteen, in hostels. Some of that will be found in histories of special education.[7] What will not be found there is the naturalistic representation of the techniques of surveillance employed by the 'sex police' and the methods of evasion employed by the underground resistance among the pupils.

But *The Panopticon* attempts more than naïve naturalism. I think of it as 'imaginary history'. It attempts to represent the historical situation of blind, perhaps all, disabled young people in residential special schools in the 1950s. This takes the form of a dramatic confrontation, which is fictional in the sense that the action represented in chapters ten and eleven never happened. There, the story of Douglas and Louise departs radically from the biography of Fred and Etta. The fictional couple take control of their own bodies by using contraceptive techniques of the time. *We* did not do this. They are caught at it by the sex police and condemned to expulsion. It was a fate *we* dreaded, but thankfully avoided. They escaped punishment by effectively challenging the rules and ideology of the carceral institution, something *we* never attempted.

As I see it, imaginary history allows us to do something that naïve naturalism cannot: namely, to pose the questions, 'Did it have to be like that and, if so, why?' Each reader will respond for him- or herself in his or her reading of the denouement, which works out issues explored in the preceding nine chapters: the mission of the school, its post-Victorian culture and the contradictions of power-knowledge.

For myself, I think of my ideal reader's response in something like the following terms. Objectively speaking, the RBS regime did not have to be like that. As the novel shows, contraceptive technique was well developed and well understood. Douglas and Louise learn about it from the well-known manual, *The Sex Factor in Marriage*, published in 1930 and reproduced in braille by the National Institute for the Blind.[8] There was, therefore, potential for personal counselling along the lines of safe sex and responsible relationships.

Why was it impossible for the authorities at RBS to institutionalise such practices in the 1950s? An obvious answer will spring to mind. They stood *in loco parentis*.[9] Parents of the 1940s and 1950s would have been no more enthusiastic for sexual permissiveness than those authorities themselves. However, such a reply is of limited value as explanation. The guards who ruled over Craigmillar were no *mere automata*, unthinkingly obeying orders.[10] They had their own values and traditions, perhaps shared by many parents. It is the task of the cultural historian to go below the surface and analyse these. To do this we must evaluate the Foucauldian theory of power-knowledge and of the asylum, or 'carceral' institution, that rested upon it. But theory, as E. P. Thompson taught us, is not to be accepted naively, and an explanation must take into account the historical facts, which Foucauldian theory does not reach.[11] It is to these historical facts that I now turn.

History and theory

First there is the issue of the 'power-knowledge' deployed in my novella by 'Major Royle', the real-life Charles H. W. G. Anderson (1900–65), head of RBS from 1932 until he died. He had been heard to say: 'I am the leading expert on the education of the blind in Scotland today.' We mainstreaming radicals in the 1970s and 1980s looked upon such claims very sceptically. Yet, his 'expertise' bore some logical relation to the situation of blind and visually impaired youngsters in Scotland at that time. Briefly, the higher professions (the Kirk or Church partially excepted) were closed to blind people. Even mainstream school teaching and clerical employment in the public service were thought to be impossible for any but the least-impaired among the partially sighted. But a labour market had expanded during the Second World War which could be penetrated by blind people and those with low vision, given appropriate training and support. It offered jobs in telephone switchboard operating, shorthand typing, welfare work as a 'home teacher' of braille and crafts, and light engineering.

The jewel in the crown of this new labour market was physiotherapy.[12] In *The Panopticon*, the narrator is Douglas's home teacher, who explains that entry into this labour market required a standard of education which local schools for the blind did not offer. None provided secondary education for those over sixteen years of age, nor impairment-specific training in telephony or shorthand typing. Charles Anderson's solution was to promote a single residential school, sufficiently well resourced, to provide these facilities, and, given the numbers involved, it had to be coeducational.

The school in which he pursued this strategy, Craigmillar, the fictional 'Craigton Hall' of my novella, had existed since 1875. At first, it served Edinburgh and the surrounding district and acquired an international reputation under William M. Stone, its headmaster from 1905 to 1932. Teachers and former pupils remembered its culture in my time as heavily Victorian. Boys and girls were not allowed to mix informally at any time, inside the school or outside in the grounds. Taking over as head in 1932, Charles Anderson transformed Craigmillar into the national school for the blind in Scotland. He was given his opportunity by reforms in Scottish education from 1936 and by the social dislocation of the Second World War. Evacuation closed local special schools and specialised units for blind children in mainstream schools, which had both coexisted with RBS since the 1880s. After the war, the former either failed to reopen or dwindled away, and RBS recruited the students they lost.

Before and after the war, reforms made provision of senior secondary education compulsory for all visually impaired pupils. They also required that training for employment be made available. In Scotland it was thought that the special schools, rather than a separate, dedicated training centre, should provide this. The enlarged RBS was better placed to claim this responsibility than the local blind schools with their tiny rolls and limited resources. Consequently, by the 1950s, residence at RBS was the only option for post-sixteen education and vocational training for blind people in Scotland, and, given the low incidence already mentioned, it had to remain coeducational.

Anderson and his fictional counterpart, Major Royle, were also conscious reformers of the domestic arrangements at RBS. Anderson sought to mitigate the extreme repression of 'the Stone age' while protecting the reputation of the school and its teenage pupils. Boys and girls could meet under supervision at organised dances, at library evenings and informally for a short time in classrooms after school. But the slightest sign of intimate contact was put down with a heavy hand. The severe repression which accompanied this liberalising policy is represented in my novella. The 'sex police' really did patrol the building and the grounds, keeping everyone under surveillance and employing the threat of expulsion. 'You'll be seen,' was the caution we always gave each other whenever we were tempted to transgress.

Thus, an educational strategy which genuinely aimed to, and did, enhance the life chances of many pupils, clashed with the natural needs of young people after puberty. This had probably been a less pressing problem for the local blind schools where the children lived at home and left school by sixteen. But the Scottish education authorities were persuaded that all blind children needed education to age eighteen, and, with vocational training added on, many attended RBS until age nineteen or twenty. It was simply not realistic to believe that all the prisoners would internalise the rules of the guards. Foucault's theories, then, require considerable qualification when applied to the historical RBS. His notion of power-knowledge allows nothing for the enhancement of some blind people's life chances that education and training could provide. Moreover, if his theory of the carceral institution seems at first sight to fit well with what I call the intimate history of Craigmillar, it must be applied here also with qualification. First, it should be noted that the official policy was undermined to some extent by the conduct of younger teaching and care staff. Some of them turned a blind eye, or even smiled indulgently on love between teenagers. In this way, the pupils came to know that the rules were not held in universal respect. Foucauldian theory seems to make such regimes too monolithic.

Respect was also undermined from the opposite angle, as it were. There was a sinister double standard at work. This was the prevalence of a certain level of sexual abuse on the part of male staff, teachers and carers towards the older pupils, both female and male. The Panopticon's plot turns on this. It is not entirely fictional, though I do not intend here to go into historical detail. Instead, I wish to underline the point that such conduct also tended to undermine respect for the unrealistic standards demanded of the pupils and therefore to encourage their underground resistance.

It should also be understood that RBS was not literally a prison, a secure, enclosed space. The pupils were not shut in. The great gates stood wide open at the end of the drive. Anyone could run away and a few did. At age sixteen, moreover, all pupils went to live outside in one of the two hostels. These were segregated by sex, and neither sex never entered the other's hostel. However, we could come and go, and no one asked where we were going or with whom. Pupils, like Etta and me, made dates and walked out to the nearby Blackford Park.

Despite these qualifications, I wish to argue that the institution was 'carceral' in the sense that the pupils were shut in psychologically. They were kept in ignorance of new developments taking place in British culture. Among these were the intimations of the sexual revolution. *The Panopticon* alludes to several manifestations: the *Daily Mirror* strip cartoon character Jane, who frolicked with the troops in risqué situations; the 1950 series run by *Picture Post*, entitled 'Sex and the Citizen'.[13] The latter frankly discussed pre-marital sex and the different mores of other cultures. Because I could see until past fourteen, I was aware of these developments. An avid reader, I had access to popular culture in the form of newspapers and magazines, which my parents brought into their home. I was also an avid consumer of motion pictures. I went blind just too early to see Marilyn Monroe, but I did see the film *Bitter Rice* (1949), with its frank representation of extra-marital sex among the proletariat of the Italian rice fields.[14] By contrast, blind pupils who were resident in RBS from early childhood to age eighteen had little or no knowledge to counter the post-Victorian culture of the place. Print media was available only in heavily edited and abridged braille versions. Even access to the radio was restricted, and the cinema screen was difficult to see for most partials.

As I have suggested, all this is prone to receive 'natural' explanation in terms of the values and technologies of the time, but there is more to be said than that. RBS had evolved from an eighteenth-century charity which became The Royal Blind Asylum and School. The 'institution' ran workshops as well as the school and still functioned under that name when I was at Craigmillar. Although sheltered employment and special education were by then conducted on separate sites, something of the asylum aura hung over the school. In *Madness and Civilisation* Foucault gives an account of the 'birth of the Asylum', which, with appropriate changes, highlights the character of the regime at RBS from the 1930s to the 1950s.[15]

First, there is the humanist episteme, which represented the asylum of the nineteenth and twentieth centuries as belonging to that 'happy age when madness was finally recognised and treated according to a truth to which we had too long remained blind'.[16] For 'asylum' read RBS and for 'madness' read 'blindness'. The discourse of the humanist episteme is well documented in the secondary literature on special education. This dated from the late eighteenth century when reformers in Paris, Liverpool and Edinburgh began to promote schools and asylums for education and industrial training. The deprivations of blind people were no longer seen as tragic afflictions of fate or punishment for sin. Instead they were the natural consequence of sense impairment. Such impairment was understood as extremely handicapping, but its effects could be more or less mitigated by appropriate instruction.

Secondly, this impairment came to be recognised as work for a new kind of expert. 'The qualified teacher of the blind' was trained to teach blind people to use their remaining senses to gain rational understanding of the world around them. By definition, such expertise was not available in other institutions of socialisation such as family, school or work-place, which were sites of danger that could do harm to any blind individual left in their charge. To have any hope of gaining a place in the human community, the blind must be treated as different, and separated from these normal institutions.

As Foucault emphasised, the asylum was to function as a surrogate family and the inmates had to be treated as minors so long as they remained.[17] As we have seen, this could be a very long time at RBS, from age two to twenty. The head was *in loco parentis* until pupils reached eighteen, although the legal age of marriage without parental consent in Scots law was sixteen. Moreover, those who left and went to the sheltered workshops were not entirely liberated from pupillage. We find this brief entry in the records of the Royal Glasgow Asylum for the Blind in 1904: 'The Managers view with disapproval marriage between two blind persons; and no such union is permitted without their consent.'[18] The records of the Royal Blind Asylum and School show that, as late as the 1950s, eugenic concerns, though weakened, were not extinct. Employees in the Edinburgh workshops who wished to marry had to submit themselves to a medical opinion regarding the possible genetic consequences.[19]

Charles Anderson was a convinced champion of the asylum principle. For corroboration of this we can now turn to historical documents. There is, for example, the record of his participation in the first International Conference of Educators of Blind Youth. It took place in 1952, a few months before I entered his school. He chaired a session on 'The Social Needs and Training of the Pre-School Blind Child.'[20] Harriet Totman, a visiting teacher of the blind in Ohio, made the lead presentation. Totman stated: 'The residential nursery for blind pre-school children has never been very popular in our country.'[21] She said it was better for well-adjusted development that the child should remain in its own home, with loving parents supported by visiting teachers. By contrast, RBS had a residential nursery which took blind children from age two. As a matter of policy, the home teachers, who were employed by the local Missions to the Outdoor Blind, but trained at RBS, were used to influence parents into surrendering their infant children to the nursery at Craigmillar. Where housing was judged to be good, parents might successfully resist handing over their children, but the episteme worked to ensure that this was regarded as exceptional.

Anderson's introductory remarks as chair of the session are highly revealing of what was involved in all this:

> I would respectfully remind you that we have not come here to negotiate or to criticise; we have come to contribute. Each country must judge what is right for the children of its people. In those countries that are thickly populated and where housing may not be good, one solution may be better than another. In those countries where life is simple and the family still holds its place, a second solution may be right.[22]

It is impossible to miss in Anderson's remarks the post-Victorian fear of physical and moral 'deterioration', of over-population and working-class slums, reinforced by a nostalgic myth of the pre-industrial past. This fear is echoed in his Annual Report on RBS in the session 1950–51:

> The class arrangements in a school for blind children most closely resemble those of the now vanishing country school where a class is a group of children working under the guidance of a teacher, but at varying stages. Fortunately, it is possible to organise the school with classes as small as a dozen to fifteen, and so children have the advantages of both class and individual education. Like the country school, Craigmillar Park is an all-age school; after Nursery and Primary Departments, the older children receive either a Junior Secondary or a Senior Secondary education, according to their ability, aptitude, and temperament, those children who require it being prepared for the University Preliminary Examination or, possibly, the Scottish Leaving Certificate.[23]

Thirdly, as Foucault saw, this kind of language masked the fear which was 'considered … of great importance' in the management of the inmates.[24] Despite its episteme of benevolence, the asylum kept inmates under constant surveillance. In this way, most could be brought to obedience without the threat of physical punishment so characteristic of earlier ages. One of the earliest heads of RBS, W. H. Illingworth, confirms that Craigmillar was indeed run on Benthamite principles:

> In Britain many of the blind schools have now adopted the class-room system, one class being separated from another by a glazed partition, so that the principal can exercise a direct supervision over the whole. By this system, also, two blind teachers and three seeing make an excellent staff for five classes, the seeing teacher being able to call his blind colleague's attention to any misconduct or eccentric movement on the part of any member of his class. Such an arrangement has proved very successful in many British schools.[25]

As my *Panopticon* shows, the transparency of glazed doors and windows was still, in the 1950s, essential to the maintenance of discipline by the staff at RBS. I was not aware of these historical records when I penned my fictional representation of Craigmillar and its head Charles Anderson. I drew upon my own experience, but it led me unerringly to the core of his beliefs, which stamped upon his school the 'carceral' regime the novella describes:

> He stood up and walked over to one of the high windows of his office. It looked out on to the wide expanse of lawn at the front. Two great elms stood like sentries in the dense shrubbery that screened it from the street. 'I've always thought of the school as a haven,' he mused. 'An asylum to shelter the vulnerable – a conservatory, where the sturdier plants can flourish and be hardened off for life outside.'[26]

Conclusion

What, then, is the bearing of *The Panopticon* on the historiography of special education? It is striking that, with one exception, histories of education of the blind afford little or no information on the quality of life experienced in them by the 'inmates'.[27] Here and there we catch a glimpse of the regime impacting upon their emotional lives. A reference in Pritchard is suggestive. The records of Liverpool School of Industry for the Blind show that, in 1800, George Eaton, a minor, 'declared his determined resolution to be married to Elizabeth Jones, also a minor, and could not be dissuaded'.[28] He was discharged. Iain Hutchison has identified similar practices by the Edinburgh asylum in the early nineteenth century.[29]

The rigid segregation of the sexes was surely a fact in the minds of workers in Scottish blind asylums when they presented their evidence to the Royal Commission on the Blind in 1889.[30] 'The rule and the strict discipline observed in these schools,' they stated, 'is an objectionable feature in the training and the upbringing of the juvenile blind'.[31] These workers, some of whom would have been educated at Craigmillar, firmly stated their preference for blind children staying at home to attend ordinary schools in their own locality. This was then common practice in Glasgow and the west of Scotland, and the Royal Commission recommended it in its report. In the early 1900s, however, central government policy began to tilt the balance towards education in residential 'institutions'.

The exception mentioned above is Sally French's oral testimony-based *History of Education of Visually Impaired People*. The stories of former pupils of residential special schools, from the 1920s on, voice repeated complaints about rigid segregation of the sexes and about the harm many felt this had done to their personal development. In his disdain for conventional historical method, Foucault thought that the recovery of the inmates' experience was impossible. The subjects of power-knowledge were hidden from history. We could know of them only 'archeologically,' digging up evidence from underground by decoding the reports of their jailers.

I wrote *The Panopticon* partly to demonstrate that this need not be true. To a large extent, it is oral history written down in fictional form. It amplifies the testimony of French's witnesses in its detailed account of the underground resistance. Moreover, it suggests the basis of that resistance in the students' experience. Sex, even in its pre-revolutionary restraints, was recreational. It compensated for the sheer boredom of so much that passed for education in the asylum: the sense of isolation from family and friends back home; the slow teaching which prolonged the years of effective 'minority'; the tedium of evenings and weekends when nothing would happen for anyone who was unwilling to join the Scouts or Guides, or play endless games of football and cricket. For us, love lightened a monotonous life, very much as it had for Robert Burns in other circumstances. Ironically, as *The Panopticon* shows, Craigmillar filled our hearts with delight in his version of romantic love:

> It was upon a Lammas night,
> When corn rigs are bonnie,
> Beneath the moon's unclouded light,
> I held awa to Annie;
> The time flew by, wi' tentless heed,
> Till 'tween the late and early,
> Wi' sma' persuasion she agreed
> To see me thro' the barley.
> The sky was blue, the wind was still,
> The moon was shining clearly;
> I set her down wi' right good will,
> Amang the rigs o' Barley.
> I kent her heart was a' my ain;
> I lov'd her most sincerely;
> I kissed her owre and owre again,
> Amang the riggs o' Barley.[32]

We sang these verses with gusto and they inspired our resistance.

One final point. French's witnesses suggest that residential school regimes began to loosen up in the 1960s as the sexual revolution gathered pace. Moira Meek, head of RBS from 1988, informs me that:

> I joined the staff in 1967 and rose through the ranks, finally retiring in 1995. I had taught pupils from P1 to S4 in 'mainstream', spending most time in what were called Junior Secondaries in troubled city housing schemes. Teaching was the only job I ever wanted to do, and the post at RBS seemed a reasonable challenge.

Although I know much of the picture you paint, I arrived when ... slow change had started. I was taken aback by much that I encountered, but each year brought new staff and new ideas. Many changes were delayed until older care staff left. When I left, we had mixed hostel accommodation, single rooms in the school, considerable parental involvement, no weekend residents, etc, etc. Maybe you and Etta would actually have enjoyed it![33]

I agree. But with one reservation. Other feedback to me suggests that the loosening may have been temporary in some respects. Health and safety legislation today makes it somewhat difficult for pupils in residential schools to get time together without surveillance.

Notes

1 I wish to thank Moira Meek, head of the Royal Blind School, Edinburgh from 1988 to 1995, and Julie Fardell, one of her successors, who as the current head read an early draft of this chapter and made valuable comments. A similar service was performed by Richard Hellewell, CEO of Royal Blind (formerly Royal Blind Asylum and School [RBAS]). I am grateful to him for this and for opening the archives of RBAS for my inspection.

2 S. French, *An Oral History of the Education of Visually Impaired People: Telling Stories for Inclusive Futures* (Lampeter: Edwin Mellen Press, 2006).

3 F. Reid, *The Panopticon* (2006) published online at www.fredreid.co.uk. A hard copy is available for consultation in the 'Papers of Dr Fred Reid' at the Modern Records Centre, University of Warwick.

4 M. Foucault, *Madness and Civilisation: A History of Insanity in the Age of Reason* (New York, NY: Vintage Books, 1988).

5 J. Bentham, *The Panopticon Writings*, ed. M. Božovič (London: Verso, 1995), p. 29.

6 S. Szreter, and K. Fisher, *Sex Before the Sexual Revolution: Intimate Life in England 1918–1963* (Cambridge: Cambridge University Press, 2010).

7 For example, see J. M. Ritchie, *Concerning the Blind* (London: Oliver & Boyd, 1930).

8 H. Wright, *The Sex Factor in Marriage* (London: Williams & Norgate, 1930).

9 *In loco parentis*, Latin, 'in the place of a parent'.

10 *Mere automata*, Latin, 'beings or individuals who act or react in a mechanical way'.

11 E. P. Thompson, *The Making of the English Working-class* (London: Gollancz, 1963).

12 Ministry of Labour and National Service, 'Report of the Working Party on the Employment of Blind Persons' (London: Ministry of Labour and National Service, 1951), paras 21–8.

13 D. J. Marcou, *All the Best: Britain's Picture Post Magazine*. Online book (1993), accessed 25 January 2015.

14 *Bitter Rice* (*Riso Amaro*) directed by Giuseppe De Santis (Lux Film, 1949).

15 Foucault, *Madness and Civilisation*, ch. 9.

16 *Ibid.*, p. 241.

17 *Ibid.*, pp. 253–4.
18 T. Stoddart, 'The history of the Royal Glasgow Asylum for the Blind', reprinted from *The Blind*, 40:175, July 1904.
19 Royal Blind Asylum and School (hereafter RBAS), Annual Reports.
20 International Conference of Educators of Blind Youth, 'The Education of Blind Youth: Proceedings of the International Conference of Educators of Blind Youth held at Bussum, Netherlands, July 25–August 2, 1952', pp. 36–52. Available from the Internet Archive at https://archive.org, accessed 25 January 2015.
21 *Ibid.*, p. 39.
22 *Ibid.*, p. 36.
23 RBAS, Annual Report 1950/51.
24 Foucault, *Madness and Civilisation*, p. 245.
25 W. H. Illingworth, *History of the Education of the Blind* (London: Sampson Low, Marston and Co, 1910), p. 163.
26 Reid, *The Panopticon*, ch. 11.
27 French, *Oral history of the Education of Visually Impaired People*.
28 D. G. Pritchard, *Education and the Handicapped, 1760–1960* (London: Routledge and Kegan Paul, 1963), p. 19.
29 I. Hutchison, *A History of Disability in Nineteenth-century Scotland* (Lewiston: Edwin Mellen Press, 2007), pp. 310–3.
30 British Royal Commission on the Blind, Deaf and Dumb, Etc. of the United Kingdom. 'Report of the Royal Commission on the Blind, Deaf and Dumb, Etc. of the United Kingdom London, 1889' (London: Eyre and Spottiswoode, 1889).
31 T. Cole, *Apart or a Part? Integration and the Growth of British Special Education* (Philadelphia, PA: Open University Press, 1989), p. 23.
32 R. Burns, *Complete Poems and Songs of Robert Burns* (Seattle, WA: CreateSpace, 2015), pp. 34–5.
33 Moira Meek, personal interview with the author, 30 July 2012.

10

ALLOWED TO BE IDLE: PERPETUATING VICTORIAN ATTITUDES TO DEAFNESS AND EMPLOYABILITY IN UNITED KINGDOM SOCIAL POLICY

Martin Atherton

Despite the plethora of social policy legislation introduced in the United Kingdom in the late twentieth century, deaf people still find themselves facing serious challenges in finding employment opportunities that match both their aspirations and their abilities. As an abundance of research from the 1990s onwards has shown, deaf people are both unemployed and under-employed at rates that would be deemed unacceptable among the general working-age population.[1]

One of the main reasons for this is that deafness is regarded as a disability in both legislative and practical terms, with the consequence that negative perceptions of disabled (and, by extension, deaf) people often influence attitudes among employers and legislators.[2] This understanding of deafness as being disabling may not necessarily be a conscious one, but the underlying message is that deaf people are disabled and so are not capable of doing a job fully or competently. Consequently, deaf and disabled people who find themselves unemployed would appear to be treated more leniently when claiming benefits and financial support, even under the increasingly draconian measures introduced as part of the United Kingdom (UK) government's financial austerity programme of the second decade of the twenty-first century. In essence, deaf people – through their legislative status as being disabled – are one of the very few groups within society who are allowed to be unemployed without some form of official censure.

This chapter will explore the current state of deaf employment in the UK and investigate the perceptions of deaf people themselves towards their employment prospects. Deaf people want to be productive members of society rather than recipients of welfare who are subjected to derogatory attitudes and expectations.[3] This examination will show how attitudes to deafness and deaf people inhibit their long-term goals to gain rewarding jobs and careers that make the best use of their abilities. The range of legislative measures that apply to deaf people will be unpacked in order to show how societal values and perceptions are both reflected and perpetuated by government policies and practices. These policies are meant to remove, rather than institutionalise, discriminatory practices in the work-place and beyond, but often fail in this objective.

The chapter will conclude by proposing the argument that current UK disability legislation is predicated on statutes and perceptions dating back to at least the early nineteenth century. The underlying principles of the 1834 Poor Law Amendment Act in England and Wales have remained embedded in virtually all subsequent measures aimed at responding to unemployment, establishing the Victorian philosophy that the vast majority of people who are out of work find themselves in this condition through choice, often as a result of their inherent indolence. One of the rare exceptions allowed by this philosophy were people whom we would now regard as disabled. The origins of contemporary attitudes towards this section of society, and the specific effects these have had on deaf people in the work-place, will be explored.

Current employability issues among deaf people in the UK

A cross-disability report jointly commissioned by Action on Hearing Loss, the Royal National Institute for Blind People, Mencap, MIND and Scope was published in 2013. It showed that government policies towards employment opportunities for disabled people were failing:

> Over half of all working-age disabled adults are unemployed, the majority of whom want to work but current approaches to lowering this figure are ineffective ... Only 46 per cent of working-age disabled people are in work, compared with nearly 80 per cent of the wider workforce ... The impact of the lack of support on disabled young people is clear: 42 per cent are not in employment, education or training (NEET), compared with 18 per cent of their non-disabled peers.[4]

In 2012, Action on Hearing Loss (previously known as the Royal National Institute for Deaf People – RNID – and the largest organisation working for deaf people in the UK) claimed that there were 135,000 people of working age with a severe to profound hearing loss.[5] These deaf people find themselves in a similar position to other disabled people in that they are more likely to be unemployed and under-employed than the general population, as demonstrated in a number of research projects and reports conducted since the 1990s.[6] In 2006 the RNID found that 37 per cent of deaf people of working age were unemployed, while similar research by the Scottish Council on Deafness (SCoD) found that deaf people in Scotland were four times more likely to be unemployed than non-disabled people.[7] The low numbers of deaf people in many areas of work suggest that deaf people are being denied employment opportunities because of what their deafness represents to employers rather than due to any inherent lack of skill or ability.

Among deaf people who have found work, frustration and a lack of job satisfaction are regularly reported. More than half of the RNID sample were of the opinion they had been held back from promotion or developing their careers primarily because of their deafness. This was also seen as the main factor in the lack of career progression among 75 per cent of the Scottish respondents. This factor, together with a lack of adequate communication services, was given as the reason for the prevention of more than half of those in the Scottish survey from pursuing further training or education. A third of the RNID sample felt that their jobs failed to make full use of their qualifications, and consequently they felt themselves to be under-utilised by their employers.

Workplace relationships were often cited as unfulfilling and unrewarding, with deaf workers having little or no social interaction with their hearing colleagues, either inside or outside work. More than half of the Scottish deaf workers interviewed felt unable to communicate with hearing co-workers, while 75 per cent of RNID respondents felt that deaf awareness training would improve their working lives by giving hearing colleagues a greater insight into the issues they faced on a daily basis.[8]

Of greater concern was the 26 per cent of deaf workers who reported facing harassment at work because of their deafness, despite such action being explicitly confronted by both disability and employment legislation. So, the overall situation for deaf people seeking employment appears to be one of limited job opportunities with little prospect of advancement or career progression. They reported working with, and for, people who know little about the reality of deaf life and whose opinions are coloured both by government policies that explicitly apply a disability label to deaf people and by mass-media representations of all disabled people as tragic figures bravely battling against their perceived afflictions. Deaf workers are likely to have little or no informal interaction and socialisation with their hearing counterparts as a consequence of the limited communication between the two parties. As a result, work is a lonely and isolating experience with few psychological or sociological rewards.[9]

Ten years after the 2006 RNID survey, the Totaljobs online employment agency revisited the employment and employability prospects of deaf people in conjunction with five national deaf charities and an extensive range of local welfare groups.[10] Their findings broadly matched those of the previous studies by Action on Hearing Loss and the SCoD, indicating little, if any, progress over the previous decade. Of the Totaljobs sample, 67 per cent earned less than £30,000 per annum, 62 per cent were still reporting discrimination from colleagues and 64 per cent felt that they had been discriminated against on the grounds of their deafness, either when applying for jobs or when seeking promotion. Of the same sample, 72 per cent claimed that they had received no specific help in finding a job as a deaf person and more than half felt that their employers had made no adjustments to meet the particular needs of their deaf employees. Almost one in five (19 per cent) of deaf employees chose not to declare their deafness when applying for jobs as they felt that this would hinder their prospects, and one interviewee reported having the job offer withdrawn when he told the employer that he was deaf.

When deaf people do find rewarding employment, there is evidence to suggest that these opportunities are often restricted to a narrow range of jobs, and that deaf people themselves tacitly support the notion that they are capable of doing only certain kinds of work. Almost 45 per cent of the Totaljobs survey participants worked in four employment sectors: healthcare, education, third sector and social care. When taken in conjunction with the salary figures cited earlier, this indicates that the majority worked in low- to middle-status roles. Tyrone Woolfe's 2004 research found that many deaf people in the UK follow one of three employment routes: they work for deaf organisations, they run their own businesses or they are unemployed and on long-term social security benefits. There is an expectation, even among deaf professionals, that they will work in deafness-related professions and settings. So, for example, deaf counsellors will largely work with deaf people, and those with media qualifications will work on deaf-related publications and programmes.[11]

As many as 8 per cent of the RNID survey of deaf people were self-employed, and here a similar picture of 'deaf working with deaf' is found.[12] Woolfe claims that self-employed deaf people predominantly provide services to other deaf people, with many not working for hearing clients at all.[13] For some, this is a matter of choice in that they prefer to work within – and support – a community and environment in which they are not seen as lacking or disabled. It can be argued that deaf people, especially sign language users, are best placed to provide services to people from a similar background, and that in such cases they provide much-needed positive role models and culturally appropriate services. However, there can also be negative consequences of focusing solely on serving a deaf clientele. Those deaf people who only work with other deaf people might be seen to perpetuate the notion that deaf people are in need of help and must be cared for by others, even if those others are themselves deaf. Deaf people in such situations, whether acting as service providers or service users, are also effectively isolating themselves from mainstream work and society rather than being fully integrated and accepted as equals in the full range of employment and careers opportunities.

Those in Woolfe's third employment category, deaf people who end up on long-term benefits, find themselves in that situation through a combination of factors. These include inadequate formal education, which leads to lack of access to higher-level qualifications, a lack of job opportunities – in particular, well-paid career structures – and a lack of awareness of the ways in which the benefits system and the wider social policy agenda in the UK regard and respond to the needs of deaf and disabled people. Assessment of a disabled person's ability to work occurs only at age eighteen, although benefits can be claimed from age sixteen. By eighteen, many young deaf people will have been institutionalised into a benefits culture, reinforced by both societal and their own negative percep-tions of deaf people's employment prospects. When this is coupled with a lack of positive role models, it is perhaps understandable why remaining on benefits might seem more attractive than taking a low-paid, low-status job.

Despite this bleak picture, deaf people can be found in a wide variety of jobs and careers and in all levels of the workforce, but for sign language users the options are much more restricted.[14] The main cause of this is the lack of support to overcome the communication barriers that exist between deaf and hearing colleagues. This is despite the funding available through Access to Work to provide such support, which is highlighted later in this chapter. The sense of isolation reported among all deaf employees in both surveys is exacerbated for sign language users, for whom access issues and being able to convince employers of their suitability for a range of jobs involving contact with the general public remain deeply problematic.

While there are some situations where not employing a sign language user would seem acceptable, for example for work in a telephone call centre, there are numerous other situations where adjustments to working practices could be made that would allow deaf people to perform these roles. As an example of the feasibility of adjustments, the international coffee chain, Starbucks, has recruited deaf sign language users at branches in Canada and Malaysia. Customers write their orders on a menu card and each customer is then given a number that appears on a screen when the order is ready. In other outlets, staff members have been provided with iPads which allow staff and deaf customers to interact via Virtual Remote Interpreters. These initiatives could be easily copied or adapted to a wide range of settings to allow deaf staff to interact with hearing customers and colleagues without any obvious disruption to the working practices of employers and with minimal outlay on additional equipment. Indeed, hearing staff could use the same method of taking and delivering orders, which could be seen as an example of equality in the workplace. That the vast majority of employers have not implemented such strategies in the past, nor begun to follow the example provided by Starbucks, suggests that there is either a lack of awareness, or an unwillingness, to make similar adjustments.[15]

In their written submission to a Parliamentary Commons Select Committee on Work and Pensions, the UK Council on Deafness stated: 'Many deaf people are unable to attain employment due to the attitudinal barriers at work.' This observation illustrates a wider problem facing deaf people seeking employment, that of employers' attitudes towards taking on deaf workers. While deaf people may have various laws to stop them being discriminated against in the workplace through their official status as having a disability, they first have to secure employment, and, as the rates of deaf unemployment show, this is extremely hard for deaf people to achieve. Without sign language users in high-profile employment, the lack of opportunities to do so can, to a degree, become self-perpetuating. A dearth of role models can lead both hearing employers and deaf people themselves to believe that this is due to a lack of ability to perform such roles, restricting both opportunities and applications – a situation that Woolfe's research supports.

Social policy and deafness

The first legislative definition of disability in the UK came through the 1948 National Assistance Act, which stated that:

> A Local Authority shall have the power to make arrangements for promoting the welfare of persons ... who are blind, deaf and dumb, and other persons who are substantially and permanently handicapped by illness, injury or congenital deformity, or such other disabilities as may be described by the minister.[16]

Through the wording used in this Act, a negative perception of the abilities and potential of disabled people became enshrined in law and explicitly included those who are 'deaf and dumb'. The use of this highly pejorative term – one that has been rejected as inaccurate and insulting by deaf people for a great many years – was indicative of the underlying attitudes that prevailed. Two legal principles were established – or, in reality, perpetuated, for they had both existed in practice for a considerable period of time. First, that disabled people were both worthy of and in need of care, and that care should be provided and organised by local authorities under the direction of national government policies. Second, that all disabled people were 'handicapped' in some way and therefore unable to be active participants in 'normal' life and, by extension, to be fully productive members of society. This legislation continued the philosophy of seeing those regarded as disabled solely in terms of what they could not do, rather than recognising and responding to what they could do. All subsequent legislation has continued this philosophy to some extent and, following on from the explicit reference to deafness in 1948, established deafness as a legally recognised form of disability.

In the early years of the twenty-first century the legislation that protects deaf people's rights in all aspects of life continues to approach deafness in terms of disability. The 1995 Disability Discrimination Act helped to codify disabled people's rights in employment and access to services, with the Act's definition of disability substantially reflecting the underlying principles and concepts expressed in the 1948 Act:

> A person is disabled for the purposes of this Act if he [sic] has a physical or mental impairment which has a substantial and long term adverse effect on his ability to carry out normal day to day activities.[17]

Once again, the notion that disability, and therefore deafness, represents abnormality is enshrined in UK law. The 2006 and 2010 Equality Acts brought all anti-discriminatory legislation under the umbrella of one legislative instrument. Equality legislation implies inequality as its starting point and seeks to address these differences in a positive and affirmative way. Indeed, it has been mandatory since 2005 for all disabled people to be assessed on their ability to work, rather than on their inabilities.[18]

However, this seems to have done little to improve and enhance deaf people's job prospects as the inequality of disabled people is emphasised and changes to established working practices are highlighted to potential employers, making deaf and disabled workers seem less attractive and more problematic. Deaf people were eligible to claim benefits such as Disabled Living Allowance and Disabled Working Allowance (both introduced in 1992), while the Access to Work (ATW) scheme was set up to help meet the costs of providing equipment and human support to allow deaf people to work alongside hearing colleagues. ATW funding is explicitly intended to support disabled people in the workplace through the provision of any technological or human assistance that may be required. The titles and eligibility of these benefits are in themselves problematic and may well act as an unintended barrier to deaf and disabled people finding work as they tend to emphasise, both to those claiming these work-related benefits and their potential employers, that they are not the same as 'normal' (i.e. non-deaf or disabled) workers.

If they are employed, such workers may require changes to be made to the established working practices of the employer, and possibly even adaptations to the fabric of the premises or the purchase of specialist equipment. All such changes have to be funded, at least in part, by the employer, and so represent an additional cost as a result of taking on a deaf or disabled worker. ATW also does nothing to address the lack of informal interaction that deaf people report in their working lives as the funding does not provide support for work-based social events, or even during breaks in the working day when such bonding usually takes place.

Changes to the scheme proposed by the Conservative–Liberal Democrat coalition government in 2013 threatened to undermine the ability of deaf people to be supported in the workplace, with employers being expected to take on an increasing responsibility for funding and employing support staff. Under the government's 'Disability Confident' campaign, which has since been revised but not significantly amended following the change of government in 2015, all deaf employees who require more than thirty hours of support per week would have this provided and paid for by their employer rather than through ATW funding. This proposal caused uproar and concern among the deaf community with the Disability Now website in 2014 suggesting that this change would lead to job losses or, at best, part-time work that did not exceed the thirty-hour limit.[19]

The changes implemented in 2016 as part of 'Disability Confident' introduced what is seen as a more intrusive and draconian assessment policy, which is perceived as being focused more on reducing costs rather than on increasing the quantity and quality of support. An open letter to the UK government minister responsible for ATW provision at the time of the new measures' introduction illustrated the depth of frustration felt by many deaf people.[20] At the time of writing, this proposal had been shelved for further consideration (but not completely withdrawn), and it is clear that, in the austerity climate that has prevailed since 2010, any changes to ATW funding would be unfortunately timed. There is greater financial responsibility on employers to fund disabled workers at a time when many businesses are under severe financial stress. Therefore, the measures are likely to make deaf employees more costly to employ than their hearing colleagues.

Where do these attitudes originate?

In many respects, deaf people in the UK remain the victims of Victorian attitudes towards disability, which continue to influence the thinking behind much of the subsequent social policies and practices that have been introduced to address the needs of disabled people. In essence, deaf people, along with all others defined as disabled, are institutionally regarded as unable to undertake meaningful employment without support from the so-called 'able-bodied' world. Until the most recent changes in government policies on supporting disabled people within employment, a different level of expectations was placed on employees with disabilities than on the majority of their non-disabled counterparts when it came to finding employment and being out of work.

Introduced in England and Wales three years before Queen Victoria came to the throne, the 1834 Poor Law Amendment Act, and the principles it introduced into governmental responses to disabled people during the Victorian era, can still be seen in social policies and disability legislation today. Although the markedly different socioeconomic (and indeed religious) contexts of Scotland and Ireland saw each country introduce its own version of Poor Law legislation, the principles of the English and Welsh approach to poverty were broadly adopted, if interpreted in differing ways. Indeed, many of the wider philosophical approaches to employment (or more, precisely, unemployment) established in 1834 continue to underpin social policy across twenty-first-century Britain and Northern Ireland, particularly the concepts of the 'deserving and undeserving poor' and the principle of 'less eligibility'. In some respects, deaf people might be seen to be treated more leniently by the benefits system through their official status as disabled people, but there are much wider consequences that have resulted in the situation outlined by Woolfe and others earlier.

The remainder of this chapter will therefore examine how deaf people in the UK remain the victims of changes in governmental responses to poverty that are influenced by Victorian attitudes towards the poor and needy in society.[21] In particular, it will be argued that the effects of the 1834 Poor Law Amendment Act continue to underpin social policy towards deaf people with deleterious consequences for their employment prospects that can be seen to the present day. At heart, deaf people, through their official classification as disabled, are allowed to be 'idle' (i.e. unemployed), while other sections of society are placed under a variety of strictures in order to be eligible for unemployment benefits.

The Poor Laws in England and Wales

The duty of local authorities to care for the poor was first standardised in England and Wales on a national basis when these countries were still predominantly rural economies.[22] The 1601 Poor Law obliged parishes (Church of England parishes were an important aspect of local government, in England in particular) to provide poor relief for paupers in their area through Poor Law Boards, which consisted of local ratepayers who also funded the scheme.[23] This Act introduced a key determinant in poor relief which underpins welfare provision to this day: the distinction between those who were classed as the 'deserving poor' and those who were seen as 'undeserving'. Those who were unable to work through no fault of their own – for example the old, infirm, widows and children – were deserving, as were those who found themselves temporarily out of work due to the cyclical nature of the rural economy with its peaks and troughs of employment needs.[24] The short-term unemployed would be found work by the parish, in return for which they received support in the form of money, food or fuel until the local economy recovered, for example once labour for harvesting work was required. On the other hand, those who were capable of working, but chose not to do so, were regarded as undeserving and were ineligible for support unless they too performed some form of work in return for poor relief.[25]

Most support allowed claimants to continue to live in their own homes rather than enter workhouses, which were used as a last resort for those who were unable to maintain a home of their own. This version of the Poor Law remained in place for over 200 years, with various amendments and alterations being made in response to changing social and economic conditions. Two of these introduced important changes that were influential in later approaches to poor relief. First, Knatchbull's Act of 1723 required claimants to reside in the workhouse, where they had to perform work in return for shelter and food, and this new regime effectively became a form of punishment for the undeserving poor.[26] Gilbert's Act of 1782 took a more lenient line, restricting workhouse admission to those deserving poor who were unable to look after themselves. All other relief was provided in claimants' own homes, but neither Act was compulsory and they provided only a framework of poor relief for those parishes that chose to adopt these practices.[27]

Throughout the period known in Britain as the Industrial Revolution, large areas of England and the southern half of Wales moved from a predominantly agricultural economy to one that was increasingly industrialised and mechanised. The more liberal Poor Law in force throughout the rapid economic and social changes that took place during the late eighteenth and early nineteenth centuries soon proved to be inadequate for the needs of large urban populations. A series of trade depressions in the years around 1800 further increased pressure on the system, which was already seen to be encouraging the idle poor not to seek work and increasing the financial burden on local rate-payers.[28] As the Poor Law guardians were also the ratepayers, they had a vested interest in changing the system they oversaw. A major revision of poor relief in England and Wales was introduced in 1834 through the Poor Law Amendment Act. Although changes to public policy were also implemented in Ireland (then one national entity across the island) in 1838, and in Scotland in 1845, these were in response to different circumstances and resulted in different outcomes for paupers and are not considered here.

Known as the New Poor Law, the 1834 Act introduced the principle of 'less eligibility' into the English and Welsh system of dealing with poverty, which was aimed at forcing people into work rather than claiming poor relief. Workhouses were restructured as bleak and unappealing places that represented the absolute last refuge of only the most desperate poor. This was achieved in various ways: relief was offered at less than the lowest locally available pay and was available only to those who resided in the workhouse, where life was unpleasant and detested. All aspects of life in the workhouse were strictly regulated with inmates expected to generate income through their labour to help pay for their shelter and sustenance. Jobs were often tedious and repetitive, such as washing and dyeing old clothes for inmates to wear and picking apart old ropes to provide the raw materials to make new ones.[29] Children were often hired out to local factories as apprentices, but, as their meagre wages were paid to the workhouse overseers, they were to all intents and purposes slave labour. In effect, all but the most incapacitated of workhouse inmates had to earn their keep. This stricter regime was meant to ensure that only those who were genuinely unable to support themselves or their families would claim poor relief, and so to reduce the burden on those who had to fund the system.[30]

Workhouses once more became a deterrent for the poor, whether they were regarded as impotent or able-bodied. The impotent poor fell into one of five categories: children, the sick, the insane, 'defectives', and the aged and infirm.[31] Entering the workhouse was generally the only form of support available to paupers, where all were subjected to the same strict regime. Those capable of work performed various tasks in return for their upkeep, with a typical ten-hour working day beginning at 5.00 a.m. and requiring them to be in bed at 8.00 p.m. Thus the punishment of the indolent poor was extended to all those unfortunate enough to have no other option than the workhouse.

The consequences for deaf people of the 1834 Poor Law Amendment Act

Precisely how deaf people in England and Wales were treated under the old Poor Law is unclear, and whether they were treated as 'deserving' or 'undeserving' poor is open to some debate. On the one hand, their deafness, particularly for those classified as 'deaf and dumb', coupled with historical perceptions of deafness as a 'handicap' or impairment, would suggest that they were seen as impotent and therefore deserving. After all, no one was seen to be deaf through their own fault or choice. However, in practical terms, deafness is no barrier to performing any number of useful and productive jobs so a harsher interpretation might have seen them classed as indolent and therefore undeserving. Lees identifies three categories of paupers who were able to enter the workhouses under the new system: the able-bodied; the aged and infirm; and the insane, lunatics and idiots.[32] Deaf people could just as easily have been categorised as 'able-bodied' through their ability to perform certain types of work, but they could be classed as 'infirm' due to their deafness. Lees also notes that all but the indolent and undeserving able-bodied were seen as 'unproductive defectives' after 1834, so were deaf people more likely to be classed as defective and thus 'unproductive'?[33]

Deaf people, particularly those who could not speak – the 'deaf and dumb' – found themselves in a disadvantageous position under the New Poor Law, whether they were regarded as 'deserving' or 'undeserving'. Deaf historian Arthur Dimmock contends that, after 1834, many deaf people who could work were placed in the workhouse for no other reason than their deafness, and not because of any physical inability or unwillingness to work.[34] Workhouse records support this contention, clearly showing that deaf people (more precisely, those classified as 'deaf and dumb') came under the purview of the Commissioners in Lunacy. References to 'deaf and dumb' inmates are also found in the annual returns of lunatic inmates provided by workhouses to the Poor Law Commission, suggesting that many, if not all such workhouse residents, were seen as both defective and unproductive, and consequently considered eligible for workhouse admission solely on the basis of being deaf.[35] Those who found themselves in workhouses effectively became innocent victims of the wider changes in attitudes towards the poor and paupers, punished for their deafness rather than for being indolent.

Precise figures for the number of deaf people who found themselves in this situation are not readily available and there is a vast amount of territory that remains unexplored concerning deaf people and the Poor Law. However, there is clear evidence that deaf people found themselves in the workhouses. *The National Index of Paupers in Workhouses in 1861* is based on the 1861 Census for England and Wales and contains information on 14,216 adult paupers who were long-term residents of English and Welsh workhouses. As well as giving their names and the length of time each pauper had been resident in the workhouse, the *Index of Paupers* also gives 'the reason assigned why the Pauper in each case is unable to maintain himself or herself'. The use of 'unable to maintain' has echoes of Knatchbull's Act and may suggest that all those recorded in the *Index* were considered to be 'deserving'; there are certainly no residents who are explicitly classified as 'indolent'.

The 1861 census identified 197 workhouse residents as 'deaf and dumb', and a 10 per cent sample of the *Index of Paupers* provided by the Genuki website contains details of 23 of these deaf and dumb inmates and raises the question of why they were allowed entry into the workhouse.[36] Only five of the sample had other physical or mental conditions that would prevent them from working. These included one who was blind, two with 'defective sight', one 'cripple' and one 'idiot'; in addition, one woman was listed as being 'deaf and dumb, and having an illegitimate child'. The remaining seventeen are merely described as 'deaf and dumb', suggesting that they were capable of working. Examples of deaf people in workhouses were found from all parts of England, indicating some consistency in the way deaf people were being treated under the New Poor Law.

It must be accepted that 197 deaf workhouse residents is not a particularly large sample from which to determine wider trends, but the true figure was undoubtedly much higher as closer examination of the data collection methodology illustrates. The figures cited from the *Index of Paupers* do not represent all workhouse residents, but relate only to adults (i.e. those over sixteen years of age) who had been resident in the workhouse for at least five years. Therefore, it is virtually certain that there were a number of deaf people who were not recorded by this survey, including those who had been in the workhouses for less than five years or who were under sixteen years of age at the time of the 1861 census. Indeed, Raymond Lee suggests a much higher figure of around 1,300 deaf workhouse inmates at that time. He bases this on an 1896 source that claimed that 6.7 per cent of a curiously precise total deaf population of 19,501 were residing in the workhouses in 1861.[37]

Although these figures must be taken with some caution, it is undeniable that deaf people were being forced to enter workhouses, often for no other obvious reason than their deafness. For those recorded in the 1861 *Index of Paupers*, the length of time they had been receiving poor relief in the workhouse varied between seven and twenty-eight years. Thomas Barlow, who had been in the workhouse in Stamford in Lincolnshire since 1839, was described as 'deaf, dumb and a cripple'. This suggests that his deafness was not necessarily the only factor in his inability to support himself. However, Mary Coram of Tavistock and Caroline Fox of Sheppey had both been receiving poor relief in their respective workhouses for sixteen years, and both were described simply as 'deaf and dumb'. In the most extreme example of a deaf and dumb workhouse resident found in the 1861 *Index of Paupers*, Selina Bence of Carlton workhouse in Yorkshire had lived there for twenty-eight years by 1861, with no indication of any other factor than being deaf and dumb given to explain her presence there.[38]

Although the ages of inmates were not recorded, 'old' and 'aged' were regularly given as the reasons for individuals being admitted to the workhouse. Some of those deaf persons listed in the *Index of Paupers* may have been too old to work, but there is nothing to suggest that this was the case. This evidence therefore suggests that, over a quarter of a century after the change in the Poor Law, deaf people were still being placed in workhouses, which supports Dimmock's assertion that this was because of their deafness, rather than an inability to work. A second Parliamentary survey, conducted in 1887, showed a remarkably similar situation to that of 1861, with 1,289 paupers classed as 'deaf and dumb' being resident in workhouses and a further 586 receiving outdoor relief.[39] However, it must be acknowledged that not all deaf people were paupers or ended up in the workhouses, nor were they all ascribed the subjective (and, at the time, legally undefined) status of 'deaf and dumb'. Nevertheless, despite the misgivings of Dimmock, the number of deaf people found in workhouses in the 1861 census still represented only a small proportion of the overall deaf population as Lee's later source confirms.

There are two possible reasons why this figure is so low. First, Anne Borsay has shown that, by 1849, only 11 per cent of non-able-bodied adults in England and Wales were resident in the workhouses, with the remainder receiving outdoor relief; the 1887 statistics cited above show that deaf people were not excluded from this form of poor relief.[40] Second, it is also very possible that the deaf welfare organisations, which had emerged in the first half of the nineteenth century, had achieved some degree of success in finding gainful employment for deaf people. The foundation of these voluntary welfare bodies adds further evidence that deaf people were being treated as deserving poor, and so found themselves placed in the workhouses.

The first organised network of deaf societies appeared in the UK soon after the change in the Poor Law and these were often a direct response to the suffering that deaf people were experiencing as a result. The Institution for providing Employment, Relief and Religious Instruction for the Deaf and Dumb was founded in London in 1841, later changing its title to the Royal Association in Aid of Deaf People, with the sole aim of keeping deaf people out of the workhouses. This was achieved by setting up missions across south-east England to provide training in various trades such as printing, bookbinding and shoemaking, which allowed deaf people to pursue gainful employment and support themselves financially.[41] However, the sheer number of deaf people to be found in workhouses strongly indicates that they were seen as being 'deserving poor' on the grounds of their perceived inability to work.

Conclusion

In what ways does the 1834 Poor Law Amendment Act continue to influence attitudes towards the employability of deaf people in the UK today? Simply this: legislation aimed at improving job and career prospects for deaf people is founded on the very perceptions and notions that underpinned the formulation of the New Poor Law almost two centuries ago. Some people are considered deserving of state support when they find themselves in poverty or unemployed; others are not and are therefore regarded as undeserving. How that distinction is drawn is still based on perceptions of the ability to work: those who can work but do not take any available job are undeserving of state support, while those who are deemed physically or mentally incapable of taking on 'normal' jobs (taking the concept of 'normal' as it is given in the definition of disability cited in the 2010 Equality Act) are deserving of special treatment. For deaf people, this means a starting point of determining what they cannot do, rather than an assessment of what they can do, based on making the best use of their skills and abilities.

It must be acknowledged that employment is not the only area of government policy that disadvantages deaf people. The education system in the UK has consistently failed to provide a teaching and learning environment that meets the specific pedagogic needs of deaf pupils and students as research by Conrad, by Powers *et al.*, and by Thoutenhoofd have all shown.[42] Without proper access to the means of gaining necessary academic qualifications, it is no surprise that deaf people lag behind their hearing counterparts in finding work. For those fortunate enough to obtain employment, their perceived and official status as having a disability, first established through the Victorian application of the 1834 Poor Law, continues to hold them back in terms of advancement, training and access to the inherent benefits to be gained from social interaction with colleagues.

The current failings of the support system in place for deaf people in the workplace are clearly identified in the 2013 cross-disability report by Trotter, which found that:

> It is clear that the current approach to employment support is not working for disabled people.
>
> The overarching intention of our proposed reforms is to empower disabled people to have greater control over their own career journeys, and to improve the effectiveness of the support they receive.
>
> Supporting disabled people through careers that match their capabilities, interests and ambitions has been shown to make working lives more sustainable than simply placing individuals in any available job.
>
> Improving skills development is a vital way of widening participation in the labour market for disadvantaged groups including disabled people.
>
> Addressing the full range of barriers disabled people experience is vital for supporting their career journeys.[43]

These failures arise from the Victorian attitude towards deafness and wider disability as something to be pitied and, at best, provided for in a charitable and paternalistic way. The very fact that a number of disability organisations can make these recommendations in the second decade of the twenty-first century shows that current policies still react to disability in a 'can't do' manner rather than identifying what a deaf or disabled person can do and putting adequate support in place. The most common word found in Trotter's recommendation is 'support', and this remains the area of greatest concern, especially in light of changes in the way disabled people are meant to be given financial and practical backing within the workplace. The most recent actions of the UK government departments responsible for disabled people, especially in relation to ATW funding, suggest that there is little positive change on the horizon, even if the rhetoric is becoming more inclusive through schemes such as 'Disability Confident' which seek to place responsibility for such support on employers. Unless and until deaf people are seen as potentially productive contributors to society on their own terms, and adequately and appropriately supported in their ambitions to be gainfully employed in work that is also interesting and emotionally rewarding rather than being regarded as a burden on the benefits system, they will continue to be part of the 'idle poor', but without the previous dispensation that arose from patronising attitudes towards people with disabilities. In many respects, deaf people in the early twenty-first century are no better off than their predecessors when it comes to finding work.

Notes

1   J. Kyle, C. Thomas and G. Pullen, *Assessing Deaf People for Employment and Rehabilitation* (Bristol: Centre for Deaf Studies, University of Bristol, 1989); J. Harris, *The Cultural Meaning of Deafness: Language, Identity and Power Relations* (Aldershot: Avebury, 1995); M. Dye, *Deaf People in the Community: Demographics of the Deaf Community in the UK* (Bristol: Deaf Studies Trust, 2000); T. Woolfe, 'Employment and Deaf People: Are we moving in the right direction?' (Paper presented at the Supporting Deaf People online conference 23 August 2004); Royal National Institute for Deaf People (hereafter RNID), *Employment Blocked: The Employment Experiences of Deaf and Hard of Hearing People* (London: RNID, 2006); Scottish Council on Deafness (hereafter SCoD), 'Statistics 2010', available from www.scod.org.uk.
2   Deafness is specifically cited in the definition of disability given in the 1995 Disability Discrimination Act, which was subsequently included in the 2010 Equality Act.
3   R. Trotter, *Work in Progress: Rethinking Employment Support for Disabled People* (London: Action on Hearing Loss, Mencap, Mind, RNIB and Scope, 2013).
4   *Ibid.*, p. 17
5   *Ibid.*, pp. 18–19.
6   Kyle *et al.*, *Assessing Deaf People*; Harris, *The Cultural Meaning of Deafness*, pp. 23–6; Dye, *Deaf People in the Community*, pp. 4–5; Woolfe, 'Employment and Deaf People'; RNID, *Employment Blocked*, pp. 1–5; SCoD, 'Statistics', n.p.

7   RNID, *Employment Blocked*, p. 3; SCoD, 'Statistics', n.p.

8   RNID, *Employment Blocked*, p. 4; SCoD, 'Statistics', n.p.

9   Dye, *Deaf People in the Community*, p. 4; Woolfe, 'Employment and Deaf People', n.p.

10 Totaljobs (2017), 'Deaf Jobseeker and Employee Experiences Survey', available at www.totaljobs.com/insidejob/deaf-jobseeker-employee-report-2016.

11 Woolfe, 'Employment and Deaf People', n.p.

12 RNID, *Employment Blocked*, p. 4.

13 Woolfe, 'Employment and Deaf People', n.p.

14 RNID, *Employment Blocked*, p. 4.

15 https://news.starbucks.com/news/deaf-partners-build-careers-at-starbucks, accessed 3 August 2016; https://news.starbucks.com/news/starbucks-is-recognized-as-a-best-place-to-work-for-disability, accessed 3 August 2016.

16 National Assistance Act 1948, Part III, 29, 1.

17 Disability Discrimination Act 1995, Part I, 1, 1.

18 Woolfe, 'Employment and Deaf People', n.p.

19 Disability Now website, https://disabilitynow.org.uk/2014/02/26/access-to-work-denying-access-to-work/, accessed 3 August 2016.

20 Stop Changes to Access to Work website, https://stopchanges2atw.com/, accessed 3 August 2016.

21 M. Rose, *The Relief of Poverty* (London: Macmillan, 1972); D. Englander, *Poverty and Poor Law Reform in 19th Century Britain 1834–1914: From Chadwick to Booth* (Harlow: Longman, 1998).

22 G. E. Boyer, *An Economic History of the English Poor Law, 1750–1850* (Cambridge: Cambridge University, 1990).

23 S. King, *Poverty and Welfare in England: 1700–1850* (Manchester: Manchester University Press, 2000).

24 L. H. Lees, *The Solidarity of Strangers: The English Poor Law and the People, 1700–1948* (Cambridge: Cambridge University, 1998).

25 Englander, *Poverty and Poor Law Reform*.

26 Rose, *The Relief of Poverty*, pp. 56–7.

27 King, *Poverty and Welfare*, pp. 41–50.

28 Lees, *The Solidarity of Strangers*, pp. 28–31.

29 For descriptive narrative on workhouse-inmate life, see M. Freeman and G. Nelson (eds), *Vicarious Vagrants: Incognito Social Explorers and the Homeless in England, 1860–1910* (Lambertville: True Bill Press, 2008).

30 Englander, *Poverty and Poor Law Reform*, pp. 19–24.

31 King, *Poverty and Welfare in England*, p. 72.

32 Lees, *The Solidarity of Strangers*, p. 12.

33 *Ibid.*, p. 21.

34 A. Dimmock, 'A brief history of the RAD', *Deaf History Journal*, Supplement X (2001), 1.

35 The National Archives (hereafter TNA), MH 12/1530/366, Report of a visit made by the Commissioners in Lunacy to the Truro Poor Law Union; TNA, MH

12/4540/247, Letter from John Dobede Taylor, Clerk to the Guardians of the Bishops Stortford Poor Law Union, to the Poor Law Board.

36 Genuki website, www.genuki.org.uk/big/eng/Paupers.

37 R. Lee, *A Beginner's Introduction to Deaf History* (Feltham: British Deaf History Society, 2004), p. 71.

38 Genuki.

39 Lee, *A Beginner's Introduction to Deaf History*, p. 72.

40 A. Borsay, *Disability and Social Policy in Britain since 1750* (Basingstoke: Palgrave, 2005), pp. 103–5.

41 Dimmock, *Brief History*, p. 3.

42 R. Conrad, *The Deaf Schoolchild* (London: Harper and Row, 1979); S. Powers, S. Gregory and E. D. Thoutenhoofd, 'The educational achievements of deaf children: a literature review executive summary', *Deafness and Education International*, 1:1 (1999), 1–9; E. D. Thoutenhoofd, 'Cochlear implanted pupils in Scottish schools: 4-year school attainment data (2000–2004)', *Journal of Deaf Studies and Deaf Education*, 11:2 (2006), 171–88.

43 Trotter, *Work in Progress*, pp. 4–7.

Index

ableism 41–2
Access to Work 181, 183–4, 192
accidents 2, 21, 23–4, 44, 60, 79, 83, 128, 134, 165
Action on Hearing Loss 178–9
Acts of Parliament 122
    Anatomy Act (1832) 23
    Disability Discrimination Act (1995) 6, 183
    Dominion Lands Act (1872) *see* Homestead Act
    Education Act (1870) 111
    Education Act (1880) 111
    Education (Scotland) Act (1872) 156, 158
    Education of Blind and Deaf-mute Children
        (Scotland) Act (1890) 123n.5
    Elementary Education (Blind and Deaf Children)
        Act (1893) 111
    Elementary Education (Defective and Epileptic
        Children) Act (1899) 111
    Equality Act (2006) 183
    Equality Act (2010) 6, 183, 191
    Gilbert's Act (1782) 186
    Habitual Drunkards Act (1879) 94, 99
    Homestead Act (1872) 38, 47
    Inebriates Act (1898) 94, 96
    Knatchbull's Act (1723) 186, 188
    Mental Deficiency Act (1913) 95, 102
    National Assistance Act (1948) 6, 182–3
    Poor Law Act (1601) 185
    Poor Law Amendment Act (1834) 13, 26, 178,
        185–6, 188, 190–1
    Poor Law Amendment (Scotland) Act (1845)
        22–3, 26, 185–6
    Poor Relief (Ireland) Act (1838) 185–6
    Public Health Act (1867) 27
agency 59, 61, 63–5, 68, 132, 143, 157–8, 179
alms houses 26
alcohol 3, 8, 11, 28, 28, 30, 32, 41, 92–105, 156
Ali Ridha Pasha 42
Allen, L. M. 115
amputation 24, 126–31, 134–7, 152
anatomy 23, 74, 77, 83–5, 87, 129, 131
Anderson, Charles H. W. G. 167–9, 171–3
Anderson, Julie 74
Anderson, Peggy L 116
aphasia 11, 113–15, 117–18
Ashby, Henry 120
Association for Visiting and Aiding Permanently
    Infirm and Imbecile Children 156
Association to Aid the Deaf and Dumb 46
asylums *see* institutions

Atherton, Martin 12–13, 156
aural surgery 73–6, 79, 81–3, 85–8
autopsy *see* post-mortem

Baber, Edward Cresswell 86
Baring, Francis 51
Barnes, Colin 3
Bennett, John Hughes 24, 27
Bentham, Jeremy 166, 172
Beveridge Report (1942) 5
Bigelow, Henry 129
Black, D. Campbell 29
Blackie, Daniel 2
blindness 8, 12, 97, 111, 114, 116, 121, 146, 164–75,
    178, 182, 189
borderlands 92–7, 99–100, 102–5
Borsay, Anne 96, 190
braille 164, 167–8, 170
Braddon, Mary Elizabeth 9
Branson, Jan 86
British Association for the Advancement of Science
    111
British Empire 7–9, 12, 38–41, 44–6, 49–51, 112
British Medical Association 111
British Otology Society 85
Broca, Paul 113–14
Brontë, Charlotte 9
Brown, Callum 4
Bunting, William 157
Burch, Susan 6
Burns, Robert 32, 174
Buttercase, Alice 151–2

Cambridge, Duke of 83
census 8, 127, 166, 188–90
cerebral palsy *see* infantile cerebral paralysis
Chadwick, Edwin 31, 193
charity 2–5, 13, 22–3, 25–6, 29, 31–3, 47, 74, 76–7,
    81–2, 86, 111, 136, 146, 148, 152–4, 157,
    160, 170, 192
    see also philanthropy
Charity Organisation Society 111
Cheatle, Arthur H. 85–7
childhood 2, 4, 7–8, 11–13, 30, 40–4, 75, 77,
    79, 81, 86, 88, 92–3, 101–5, 110–23, 128,
    145–60, 164–75, 187, 189
Christie, James 149
Church Colonisation Society 48
Church Missionary Society 41–2

Church of England 185
Cleall, Esme 7, 9, 81
Clugston, Beatrice 156
Collins, Wilkie 9
colonialism 9, 38–51
  see also British Empire
Colton, Rev Calvin 136
Commissioners in Lunacy 188
Conrad, R. 191
Conservative Party 184
convalescent homes 10, 13, 110, 112–13, 143, 146,
  151–5, 157–9, 161n.46
  Cromwell House 113
  Dundonald Home 151
  Eaglesham 151
  Fresh Air Fortnight Home 151
  Ravenscraig Children's Convalescent Home
    151–4, 159, 161n.46
  Schaw Convalescent Home 153
Cox, Jeffrey 41
Crabbe, Christine 95
Craik, Dinah 9
crime 29, 82, 93, 95–8, 100–4
Cullen, William 30
Cumberland, Duke of 76
Curtis, John Harris 73–9, 81–4, 86–7

Darwin, Charles 118, 122
de Rothschild, Ferdinand 112
deaf community 6, 41, 46, 49, 184
deaf culture 6, 39, 50, 73–4, 86
deaf education 9, 45–6, 87–8
deafness 6–8, 10–13, 40–51, 55–7, 73–88, 117, 119,
  146, 152, 177–92
degeneration 11, 23, 29–30, 92, 94, 97–8, 100–1,
  104
de Tocqueville, Alexis 131
Dickens, Charles 9, 29, 67
Dimmock, Arthur 188, 190
Disabled Living Allowance 183
Disabled Working Allowance 183
Disability Confident 184, 192
Disability Now 184
disease 2, 21, 23–4, 26–7, 29, 31–2, 73–7, 84–5, 88,
  92–4, 96–101, 103–4, 112–13, 118, 122,
  131, 145–8, 151–3, 156–7
dispensaries 10, 25, 29, 73–5, 80, 82–3, 86, 112,
  148–51, 155, 157
  Royal Dispensary for Diseases of the Ear 10–11,
    73–85, 87–8
dissection 23, 27–8, 84
Douglass, Darwin DeForrest 131
Dow, Derek 149
dyslexia 114–17, 122

East India Company 40, 42, 51
East Park School 158–9

education 4, 7, 10, 13, 22, 27, 31, 39–40, 45–7, 94,
  101, 110–11, 104, 106, 119–20, 122, 156,
  158–9, 166, 173, 179, 181, 191
  blind 111, 164–75
  deaf 45–6, 74–5, 79, 88, 111, 114, 117, 119–20,
    178–81
  sex 164
  special 111, 156, 164–75
elderly 3–4, 123, 184, 188–9
Eliot, George 9, 55–9, 62–3, 65–7
emigration 9, 44, 47–8
employment 1–4, 8, 13, 47–8, 101, 119, 126–7,
  135–7, 152, 165–8, 170–1, 173, 177–92
Engels, Frederick 24, 30
Enlightenment, Scottish 30
epilepsy 41, 95, 98, 111, 122
equality 6, 181, 183, 191
Esmail, Jennifer 74
ethics 6, 25, 62, 82
eugenics 11, 73, 92, 94, 96, 100, 171

Fardell, Julie 175n.1
feeble-mindedness 92, 94–5, 102, 114
fiction 8, 39, 55–68, 164, 166–9, 173–4
Fisher, Kate 166
Flournoy, John Jacobus 48–9
Fothergill, J. Milner 29, 30
Foucault, Michel 165–7, 169–73
Franklin Institute 133
Frawley, Maria 2
Fratz, Deborah 8–10
French, Sally 164, 173–4
fresh air therapy 113, 136, 149–51, 153, 158–9
Fry, Elizabeth 47
Fry, Richenda 47
Fyfe, William Morton 158

Galton, Francis 111
Garland-Thomson, Rosemarie 135
Gaskell, Elizabeth 9, 67, 118
gender 3, 8, 11, 32, 412, 56, 61, 63, 93, 96–8, 100–5,
  127, 134, 137, 148–9, 151
Genuki 188–9
George IV, King 76, 83
Gladstone, William 48
Glasgow Poor Children's Fresh Air Fortnight 151
Glasgow Town Council 27
Goggin, Gerard 38
Golding-Bird, Cuthbert Hilton 121
Granshaw, Lindsay 74
Great Exhibition (1851) 129–31
Groom, Jane 9, 38, 40, 44–6, 49–51
Groves, Anthony 42

Hadden, Walter Bough 117, 120
Hale-White, William 121
Halford, Sir Henry 76

harassment 179
Hardy, Thomas 9
Harewood, Earl of 83
Harris, Jose 2
Harvey, William 83–7
Hay, James 4
Hellal, Paula 10–11
Hellewell, Richard 175n.1
heredity 92–8, 100, 102–3
Herschbach, Lisa 134
Hinshelwood, James 116–17, 121
Hirsch, Karen 38
Holmes, Martha Stoddard 56
hospitals 7, 9–10, 166, 186
    Alexandra Hospital for Hip Disease, London 112
    Belvedere Hospital, Glasgow 27
    Children's Home Hospital, Strathblane 154–5, 157, 159, 161n.48
    Children's Hospital of Philadelphia 146
    Evelina Hospital, London 112
    foundling 24
    Glasgow Royal Infirmary 9, 22–33, 146–7, 153, 157
    Glasgow Western Infirmary 147–8
    Hôtel-Dieu, Paris 130
    Institute for Sick Children, Dublin 112, 146
    l'Hôpital des Enfants Malades, Paris 112, 146
    Metropolitan Ear, Nose and Throat Hospital, London 87
    paediatric 110–13, 118, 122, 147–8, 151, 160–1n.9
    Royal Ear Hospital, London 11
    Royal Hospital for Sick Children, Edinburgh 146
    Royal Hospital for Sick Children, Glasgow 13, 146–59
    Royal Infirmary of Edinburgh 9, 22–33
    St Anna's Children's Hospital, Vienna 146
    St Thomas' Hospital, London 117
    voluntary 5, 8, 22–3, 25–30, 33, 157
housing 2–3, 24, 33, 99, 101, 103, 112–13, 147–9, 151–4, 156, 159, 160n.9, 162n.40, 170–2, 186
Hudson, Erasmus Darwin 128–9
Hughes, Bill 6
Hutchison, Iain 12–13, 173

Ibbotson, Margaret 60–1, 67
Illingworth, William H. 172
impairment 2, 4–10, 124, 21, 23–4, 28–30, 32–3, 39, 41, 50, 145–6, 152, 157–60, 168, 187
    linguistic 110–23
    mental 1–2, 6, 8, 145–6, 156, 170, 175, 182–3, 187–9, 191
    physical 1, 6, 8, 11, 13, 21, 111, 145, 152, 156–7, 182–3, 189, 191
    sensory 1–2, 6, 8, 11, 110–11, 145, 156, 171
    see also blindness, deafness

imperialism see British Empire
inebriation see alcohol
industrialisation 2–4, 8, 30, 100, 126, 131, 145–6, 159, 172, 186
infantile cerebral paralysis 113–14, 153, 159
insanity see impairment, mental
International Conference of Educators of Blind Youth (1952) 171
institutionalisation 2–3, 7, 10, 12, 92–9, 102, 104, 110–13, 145, 147, 159, 178, 181, 184
institutions 2–3, 7, 10–11, 13, 16, 31, 38, 50, 57–9, 65–6, 74, 77, 81–2, 93–9, 101–2, 104, 111–12, 114, 119, 121, 129, 145–6, 151, 154–8, 165–7, 169–71, 173
    Baldovan Institution for Treatment and Education of Imbecile Children 146, 156
    blind 12, 146, 156, 164, 170, 173
    British Asylum for the Deaf and Dumb 46
    Broomhill Home for Incurables 156
    deaf 44–7, 73–88, 146, 156, 190
    Earlswood Asylum 84
    East Park Home for Infirm Children 13, 146, 155–60
    Edinburgh Deaf Asylum 45
    Glasgow Institution for the Deaf and Dumb 77
    Institute for Diseases of the Ear 87
    Institution for providing Employment, Relief and Religions Instruction for the Deaf and Dumb 190
    Liverpool School of Industry for the Blind 173
    London Asylum for the Deaf and Dumb 75, 79, 81, 84
    Manchester Deaf and Dumb School 46
    mental 2–3, 156
    National Institute for the Blind 167
    Royal Blind School, Edinburgh 164–75
    Royal Glasgow Asylum for the Blind 171
    Scottish National Institution for the Education of Imbecile Children 156
Interdepartmental Committee on Physical Deterioration 100–1
International College of Otology 85
isolation 38, 59, 65, 137, 174, 179–81

Jackson, Mark 94
Jewett, Benjamin W. 131
Jewson, Nicholas 76
Jones, Claire 6
Jones, Gareth Stedman 101
Jones, Ian 5

Kafer, Alison 6
Kerr, Norman 98–100
Kings College London 85
Kitto, John 9, 38, 40–4, 46, 49–51
Kreigal, Leonard 39
Kudlick, Catherine 81, 87

Labour Party 4
Ladd, Paddy 46
Lamarck, Jean-Baptiste 29
Lane, Harlan 39
language 7–8, 11, 22, 38–9, 41–3, 61, 66, 95,
    110–23, 172
Lees, Lynn Hollen 187–8
legislation 3–4, 6, 10, 13, 47, 94–5, 103, 123, 175,
    177–9, 182–5, 190
Levine, George 66–7
Liberal Democrat Party 184
Liberal Party 4
Lieffers, Caroline 7, 10, 12
Linker, Beth 74, 94
lip-reading 120
Lister, Joseph 22
literacy 64, 115–18, 122
literature 8–9, 14, 30, 40, 55–68, 76, 114–17, 121,
    127, 130, 132, 164, 170–1
    see also publications
Little, John William 113
London Missionary Society 41
London School Board 46
Lorch, Marjorie 10–11
Love, James Kerr 77

McClelland, Michelle 103
Macewen, William 148
McGuire, Coreen 74
Mackenzie, Francis Humberstone 51
Mackie, Mrs J. L. 149
Macleod, Sir George 149
marriage 41, 60–6, 152, 171, 173
Martineau, Harriet 9, 55–67
Maryland Institute 130
Matheson, Farquhar 85
Maudsley, Henry 95–6
Maule, William 75
Maurice, Sir John Frederick 100
Medresco hearing aid 76
Meek, Moira 174–5
Meier-Hedde, Regine 116
Mencap 178
Mihm, Stephen 132
Milan Conference on Education of the Deaf (1880)
    46–8
military 9, 14, 100
Miller, Don 86
MIND 178
missionaries 9, 38, 41–3, 46
Missions to the Outdoor Blind 171–2
Mitchell, Rebecca N. 67
Mitchell, Silas Weir 135
models of disability 5–6, 10, 12, 74, 127,
    138
Montrose, Duchess of 148–9, 157

morals 1–2, 4–5, 8, 13, 29–31, 56–9, 62, 64–7, 73,
    83, 93–4, 96, 99–105, 134, 136, 172
Morel, Bénédict Augustin 98
Morgan, William Pringle 116
mortality 24, 96, 101, 146–7, 160–1n.9
Mott, Valentine 129

National Health Service 7, 76, 154, 159–60, 161n.48
National Institute for the Blind 167
National Temperance League 101
NEET 178
New Hampshire Temperance Society 133
Newell, Christopher 38
Newman, Sophia Maria 76
Noyes Jnr, Russell 28
nutrition 24, 29, 148–9, 151, 156, 159

O'Connor, Erin 134
oral testimony 177–8, 182
oralism 74, 86–8, 120, 164, 173, 174
orientalism 38, 43–4
Osler, William 113

Paget, Henry William 128
Palmer, Benjamin Franklin 12, 126–37, 175
Parliamentary Select Committee on Works and
    Pensions 182
Parry, Robert 150
Parsons, Talcott 28
passing 10, 12, 74, 133
Paterson, Kevin 6
Paterson, Margaret Montgomery 149
paupers 23, 26, 29, 97, 185–90
Pearson, Amy Farnbach 9, 157
Peel, Sir Robert 83
Percival, Thomas 25
phantom limb 135
philanthropy 3–4, 23, 26, 46, 50, 76, 81–2, 86,
    130–1, 146–9, 151–4, 156–8, 160
    see also charity
phthisis see tuberculosis
Ponsonby, Rt Rev Richard 82
poor see paupers, poor laws, poverty
Poor Law Commission 188
poor laws 1–2, 13, 22, 26, 185–91
    outdoor relief 186, 190
    poor relief 2, 26, 185–90
poorhouses 10, 23, 26, 166
Porter, Bernard 49
postcolonialism 39, 43
post-mortem 23, 27–8, 113–14
poverty 1–4, 10, 13, 21–33, 44, 46–7, 61, 75–6, 81,
    93, 95–7, 101, 104–5, 111–12, 128, 136,
    156, 160, 160n.9, 185–92
Powers, Stephen 191
prisons 98–9, 101–2, 166, 169–70

Pritchard, D. G. 173
Pritchard, Urban 85–7, 173, 176
prosthetics 6, 8, 12, 126–38, 156
prostitution 31, 97, 102
publications
  Absent-Minded Imperialists 49
  Autobiography of a Deaf Mute 45
  Bitter Rice (film) 170
  Boston Medical and Surgical Journal 135
  Cases Illustrative of the Treatment of Diseases of the
    Ear 79
  Condition of the Working-class in England, The 24
  Cyclopaedia of Biblical Literature 43
  Daily Mirror 170
  Deerbrook 56, 59–62, 66
  Essay on the origin, habits, and c. of the African race
    49
  Family Oracle of Health 75
  Future for the Deaf and Dumb in the Canadian
    North West 48
  History of Education of Visually Impaired People
    173
  History of Palestine and the Holy Land, including a
    Complete History of the Jews 43
  History of Palestine from the Patriarchal Age to the
    Present Time 43
  How to Observe Morals and Manners 57–8
  Illustrations of Political Economy 56
  International Archives of Otology 85
  Lancet, The 29, 116
  Letter to the Deaf 57, 60
  Madness and Civilisation 170
  Maintenance of Health 29
  Medical Ethics 25
  Mill on the Floss, The 56, 59, 63, 65–6
  Moral Institution Sanctioned by the Scriptures and
    the Savior 49
  National Index of Paupers in Workhouses in 1861,
    The 188–9
  New Monthly Magazine 75
  New York Daily Times 128, 130
  Our Mutual Friend 67
  Outcast London 101
  Panopticon, The 13, 164–6, 168–70, 173–4
  Penny Magazine 42
  Pictorial Bible 43
  Picture Post 170
  Punch 130, 137
  Reply to a Pamphlet Entitled, Bondage 49
  Ruth 67
  Scientific American 136
  'Sex and the Citizen' 170
  Sex before the Sexual Revolution 166
  Sex Factor in Marriage, The 167
  Studies of Childhood 122
  Times, The 99, 130, 137

Water-Cure Journal 129
'Where to Get Men' 100

quackery 73, 82–3

race 8, 38–41, 46–7, 49–50, 92, 94, 100–1, 104–5
racism 49
reformatories 93, 95–7, 101–4
rehabilitation 7, 10, 99, 101–2, 126, 192
Reid, Etta 164–5, 167, 170
Reid, Fred 12–13
religion 2–5, 30, 41–2, 46, 48, 73, 81–2, 99, 116,
    152–4, 158, 160, 168, 185, 190
Rembis, Michael 6
remediation 120–1
respectability 25, 28, 31–3, 74, 83, 97, 99
responsibility 4–5, 24, 28–31, 74, 78, 84, 86, 94,
    96–7, 101, 104, 123, 153, 167–8, 184, 192
Richardson, Rev J. 78
rickets 2, 4, 145, 147–8, 154, 157–8
Riehl, W. H. 55, 58
Risse, Günter B. 115
Rose, Sarah 3
Rosebery, Lord 100
Rowntree, Seebohm 3
Royal Association in Aid of Deaf People 190
Royal Bounty Fund 48
Royal College of Surgeons 130
Royal Commission on the Blind (1889) 173, 176
Royal Commission on the Liquor Licensing Laws
    100, 102
Royal National Institution for Blind People 178
Royal National Institution for Deaf People 178–80
Royal Navy 75–6, 154
Royal Society of Medicine 85

Said, Edward 43
Schaw, Archibald S. 153, 161n.40
Schaw, Marjory 153, 161n.40
Schmaltz, Heinrich 77
schools see education
Scope 178
Scottish Council on Deafness 178–9
sexual abuse 169
Shanks, Robert 159
Sherry, Mark 39
sign language 6, 39, 41, 43, 45, 50, 73, 180–2
Sims, John 76
slavery 38, 40, 48, 51, 56, 187
Sloan, A. Bankier 155
Smith, John 48
Smith, Rev Samuel 46
Smyth, Henry Sheppard 82–3
social class 1–4, 8–9, 11, 21–33, 41, 44, 46, 48–9,
    55–6, 58, 61, 76, 83, 93, 96–105, 130, 132,
    134, 148–50, 158–60, 172

Social Darwinism 11, 94, 100, 118
social exclusion 24–5, 33, 38, 50, 57, 59–60, 63, 101
social inclusion 26, 56, 127, 138
social policy 7, 11–13, 25, 41, 92–4, 96, 101, 104–5, 167, 171, 173, 177–92
social reform 2, 5, 8–10, 21, 24, 28–31, 33, 94, 96–8, 122, 168–9, 171, 191

Stansbury, Charles 131, 134, 136
Starbucks 181–2
Starkey, Pat 121–2
Starr, Paul 128
stereotyping 11
stethoscope 22
Stevenson, Robert Louis 9
stigma 21, 28, 30, 33, 39, 93, 97–8, 103, 126, 133
Stoker, Bram 9
Stone, Deborah 96
Stone, William M. 168–9
Stott, R. 30
Sully, James 122
surveillance 11–13, 93, 104, 166, 169, 172, 175
Szasz, Thomas 38
Szreter, Simon 166

Tait, George 9, 38, 40, 44–6, 49–51
temperance 92–4, 96–7, 100–5, 132–3
testimony 13, 127, 164, 167–8, 170
Thatcher, Margaret 5, 155
therapy 10, 98–9, 105, 117, 120–1, 165, 168
Thompson, E. P. 167, 175
Thoutenhoofd, Ernst D. 191
Tierney, Sir Matthew John 76
Totaljobs 179–80
Totman, Harriet 171
Toynbee, Joseph 82, 84
Trades Union Congress 4
training,
    medical 22, 27, 75, 128, 147, 151, 157–8
    vocational 2, 111, 158, 1689, 171, 173, 179, 191
Trinity Congregation Church 151
Trotter, Ross 191–2
tuberculosis 2, 22–5, 29, 31–2, 145, 147–8, 152–3, 157, 159

Tupper, Sir Charles 48
Turner, David 2

UK Council on Deafness 182
Universal Dispensary 112
universities
    Edinburgh 165
    Glasgow 147, 149
    Warwick 165
urbanisation 4, 14, 101, 113, 126, 128, 132, 186

Velpeau, Alfred 133–4
Veracini, Lorenzo 46
Victoria, Queen 3–4, 14, 83, 185
Victorian attitudes 185, 188, 191–2
Victorian values 5, 7, 158
Virdi, Jaipreet 10
Virtual Remote Interpreters 181

Waddington, Keir 82
Wakem, Philip 56, 59, 62–5, 67
war 5, 7, 13, 79, 153, 157, 159–60
    American Civil War 126, 132, 134
    Boer War 96, 100
    Great War, The 4, 13
    Second World War 5, 13, 151, 154, 158–9, 164, 168
Warner, Francis 119
Warner, John Harley 115
Watson, Margaret 154
welfare 4–5, 96, 179, 190
West, Charles 112–13, 119
Wheatcroft, Sue 5
William IV, King 83
Woiak, Joanne 10–11
Woolfe, Tyrone 180–2, 185
workhouses 10, 26, 41, 47, 97, 166, 186–90
Worster-Drought, Cecil Charles 115
Wright, G. A. 120
Wright, William 77
Wyllie, John 120

Yearsley, James 84, 87
Yeo, Stephen 3
Yonge, Charlotte 9
Young, Maria 56, 59–65, 67